State of Emergence

Some Other Titles from Falcon Press

STATE OF EMERGENCE

experiments in group ritual dynamics

by
Antero Alli

Preface by
Jogen Salzberg

THE *Original* FALCON PRESS
TEMPE, ARIZONA, U.S.A.

International Standard Book Number: 978-1-935150-71-8
ISBN: 978-1-61869-710-3 (mobi)
ISBN: 978-1-61869-711-0 (ePub)
Library of Congress Control Number: 2020946547

First Edition 2020
First eBook Edition 2020

Front Cover Image by James Koehnline

The paper used in this publication meets the minimum requirements of the American National Standard for Permanence of Paper for Printed Library Materials Z39.48-1984

Address all inquiries to:
The Original Falcon Press
1753 East Broadway Road #101-277
Tempe, AZ 85282 U.S.A.

(or)
PO Box 3540
Silver Springs NV 89429 U.S.A.

website: http://www.originalfalcon.com
email: info@originalfalcon.com

for Sylvi
your love, your brilliance

ACKNOWLEDGEMENTS

The work processes represented here have been significantly influenced by these extraordinary individuals, all of whom I remain eternally grateful for.

KEITH BERGER
  for early Mime training and our lasting friendship

DAVID ROSENBLOOM
  for directing the 1977 Berkeley initiatory group

SYLVI ALLI
  for your fully embodied voice and your methods

NICK WALKER, Sensei
  for your consistency of presence and integrity

JULIAN SIMEON
  for your impeccable work ethic and friendship

ROBIN COOMER
  for your resonating vocal creations and friendship

MEMORIE EDEN
  for your undying passion for performance

MAPLE HOLMES
  for your courage to keep breaking new ground

NICK THARCHER
  for your fierce loyalty to Falcon's flight

TABLE OF CONTENTS

PREFACE BY JOGEN SALZBERG
Confessions of a Zen Priest.. 13

INTRODUCTION BY ANTERO ALLI
Welcome to Post-History!... 15

ORIENTATION

PARATHEATRICAL RESEARCH
Miraculous Interactions of Self-Governing Bodies.................... 23

THE ASOCIAL CLIMATE
The Social Bypass of Paratheatrical Process......................... 32

THE RITUAL FACILITATOR
On Set and Setting, Observation and Talking......................... 36

THE METHODS

THE CRUX METHOD OF NO-FORM
Intimacy with Void; Create Trance, Break Trance.................... 43

THE FIVE INTENTIONS
Dimensionality in Source Work.. 46

TRIGGER METHODS
The Nuts and Bolts of this Ritual Technology........................ 49

EMBODIED VOICE WORK
The Unity of Sound and Movement 56

THE RITUALS

THE 5-PHASE WARM-UP CYCLE
Towards Feeling the Body Deeply................................ 61

INITIATION TO SOURCE WORK
Direct Engagement & Expression of Energies.............. 63

POLARITY WORK
The Interplay of Contraries...................................... 65

THE VERTICALITY RITUAL STRUCTURE
Difficulty Level (1 out of 5)...................................... 67

THE FOUR ELEMENTS RITUAL STRUCTURE
Difficulty Level (2 out of 5)...................................... 72

THE DREAMING RITUAL STRUCTURE
Difficulty Level (3 out of 5)...................................... 77

SAVIOR, VICTIM, PERSECUTOR RITUAL (SHADOW WORK)
Difficulty Level (4 out of 5)...................................... 83

THE MUSES RITUAL STRUCTURE
Difficulty Level (5 out of 5)...................................... 91

LAB REPORTS

PARTICIPANT EXPERIENCES
Reports from Those Who Have Done This Work.............. 101

THE EMBODIED VOICE
An Interview with Sylvi Alli...................................... 110

PEARLS & PERILS OF COURTING THE MUSES
Ritual Journal Entries, 2010–2019.............................. 117

NO-FORM REVELATIONS
It's Never What I Think... 123

POTENTIAL THREATS, DANGERS, SELF-DELUSION
Perils & Pratfalls of Long-term Paratheatrical Work.............. 127

CLOSURE

UNDOING THE WORLD
Manifesto, Parts 1–5 139

THE FRUITION OF PERFORMANCE
Towards the End of an Era 169

ABOUT THE AUTHOR 178

PREFACE
by Jogen Salzberg

CONFESSIONS OF A ZEN PRIEST

As a Zen priest during a fifteen-year residence at a Zen monastery, much of my life has been devoted to making the ego transparent and awareness spacious and receptive, for the sake of helping others find peace and tenderness in themselves. This paratheatrical work has some common ground to that and other practices I've done within Zen and Tantric Buddhism except it hits on something that is of precious import and resonance for me, something I've found nowhere else. Being = Art. Universe as Expression, the fulfillment of my existence being the range and depth and intensity of embodiment available. For no reason other than itself. In the paratheatrical work the transparency and spaciousness of no-form shapes forth as energies/selves that delight, exhilarate, humiliate, sanctify and terrify—sometimes all in one session! In these rituals, magic has flirted and the sacred has visited in ways I never expect.

This work is deepening my appreciation for the nuances of existence. Sourcing Love, I've brought to light and felt more intensely my Idealism around Love—fully present in the Innocence of that as well as the blushing revelation of its immaturity and call to be rounded out in my relationships. Serving Love's deep agony, I let the ache of that

13

vibrate my whole body and found wails coming forth from deep belly, found myself harrowed and enlivened being the servant and channel of that world-wound wail. Surrendering to Earthbody, I've been in deeper relationship to the raw animalness of body, exposing and healing a tendency to numb out from high-saturation sensitivity in my flesh and muscle. Connecting with what I love about the Dreambody, feeling the translucent colors of that source light up and move my being in so many different forms, my relationship to Dream and the Imaginal realms is much more open and post-lab; I continue to experience a clearer and wider continuum between Dream and Awake.

Spontaneity, a life element that is at the heart of why I keep on eating and breathing, is a continual theme for me in this work. I came in with the question about whether there truly is such a thing as spontaneity or whether everything is just a recombination of previous habits, impressions and experiences. Now I say: Spontaneity is real. At times I am animated beyond myself, beyond my history, beyond my fixed beliefs in this work. And I've found meaning and renewal in knowing I'm serving some cosmic imperative to give life to: ? ? ? ?, as a channel and student and body for the Universe outgrowing small, pedestrian ideas of what my life is for.

— Jogen Adam Salzberg, Sensei,
Great Vow Zen Monastery, Oregon

INTRODUCTION
by Antero Alli

WELCOME TO POST-HISTORY!

I'm writing this six months into the era of Covid here in Portland, Oregon where peaceful protests and antifa riots have owned the downtown streets every night for the past four months; it's an intermittent war zone. Terms like "quarantine" and "social distancing" are spoken and heard in hypnotic repetition without much thought about what they actually mean. I thought quarantine meant triage or separation of the sick away from the healthy, such as happens in hospitals. Yet it's presented in mass media and by governing officials as if that's what's actually happening all around the world. What's happening looks more like *voluntary house arrest* than a quarantine.

The "social distancing" thing caught my attention which looks more like *an asocial experiment* to me, something we do in paratheatrical work where everyone pays more attention to the space around themselves and around others. In paratheatrical work, there's a method called "space forming" where we redirect our attention off of ourselves and onto the space around and above us, as well as the space between others and ourselves. Space forming amplifies spatial awareness, and cultivates an asocial climate that supports an exploration of energy sources in the Body as movement resources.

15

During the Covid pandemic, the populace is being conditioned to increase spatial awareness. This seems important. The awareness of space as a value runs counter to the consumerist, materialistic mindset defined by a constant filling of space—*within our minds, in our homes, in our schedules*—with more and more things—more stuff. Losing a sense of space can lead to a wavering sense of dislocation, of not knowing where or who you truly are. This juncture in time and space feels like a crossroads of wavering discontinuity in history, as we know it—the end of democracy as we've known it, the end of money as we've known it, the end of socialization as we know it. With history in the rear view mirror and Post-history on the horizon, this interim era feels like what Tibetan Buddhists call the "bardo" realms between incarnations. The Covid bardo?

Welcome to Post-History! This paratheatrical approach to ritual is very, very old and very, very new. It initiates participants into the art of sourcing energies, or spirits, in the Body through a kind of neo-shamanic discipline of soul-making. *Read the previous sentence, again.* Over time, the somatic practice of this "sourcery" builds a kind of psychic immunity to the toxic dying cultures at large and the hypnosis of mass media. This book was written for those ready to explore novel ways of being, relating and doing through *asocial group ritual experimentation.* Those seeking a philosophy, belief system, religion or dogma might be better served looking elsewhere, such as your neighborhood churches, synagogues, monasteries, ashrams and temples.

Some or much of this book may seem abstract to those with little or no somatic, movement, dance, ritual or physical theatre-type experience. Those already swimming in these waters may recognize the terms in this book and their sometimes incomplete definitions and directions. This incompleteness is intentional. When things are too spelled out or explained, it kills the spirit of discovery to experience things for oneself. Those who require everything spelled out or explained before attempting anything new may find this book a bit frustrating. This book may not be for everybody.

In the paratheatrical process outlined in this book, the Body is presented as *the living embodiment of the so-called Subconscious mind* with its vast internal landscape of interrelated, interactive bio-systems and their autonomous forces, buried memories, emotions, sensation, images and sovereign empire of passions. When the Body can be felt deeply (see "The 5-Phase Warm-Up Cycle"), a door opens to the peaks and valleys of this interior dimension and its soulful domain of humanity, creaturehood and divinity. The ritual sources introduced in this book are assumed *to already exist within us as the existing conditions of our inner and outer lives.* There is nothing to make up or believe here. These ritual sources refer to living psychic dynamics within each of us at various degrees of depth and accessibility. The rituals are designed for accessing these depths and giving them outward expression.

The current hypermedia era, with its internet addictions and over-reliance on gadgets, diminishes the capacity for actual experience. Simulation replaces stimulation;

immediate gratification supplants the sense of immediacy. Since the primary aim of this work is *to restore the capacity for direct experience, or gnosis,* no doctrine or dogma is attached to it. There is nothing anyone needs to believe before doing this work. If there is a belief involved it would be a committed belief in oneself or more specifically, a belief in one's direct experience as *a source of spiritual authority.* But these beliefs must be earned through firsthand experience. As the capacity for experience deepens and gains breadth within us, there's simply less need for beliefs. Who needs belief when you have experience?

This book offers two levels of opportunity for active paratheatrical research: *short-term and long-term.* Short-term users can use the methods to augment and challenge whatever movement, theatre, dance or ritual practice you're already engaged in. Dip in and out of the book; use whatever works, toss the rest. All the methods and rituals here were distilled over decades of time-intensive workshops running anywhere from four to twelve weeks at a stretch, meeting once a week for three hours at a time, sometimes, two or three times a week. When performed in sequence, the five rituals in this book—from the least difficult Verticality ritual to the most difficult Muses ritual—*were designed for long-term users* who can organize a group to work over four to six weeks at a time and maybe longer. Groups of six to twelve have worked best in this medium.

State of Emergence is my third and final paratheatrical book after *All Rites Reversed: Ritual Technology for Self-Initiation* (1986; Falcon Press) and *Towards an Archeol-*

ogy of the Soul (2003; Vertical Pool). This final book distills a harvest of paratheatrical work over the past seventeen years that came to a final fruition throughout a series of five Performance Ritual productions staged between 2016 and 2018 in Portland, Oregon (see the photos at the back of this book).

As of Autumn Equinox 2019, I ceased all paratheatrical workshops and performance rituals. After forty-two years, I've been deeply fulfilled and grateful to everyone joining me on this journey; we know who we are. We had an epic run and it's time to reinvent myself, again. Though I don't see teaching any more groups in this ritual process—*never say never, right?*—I am excited by the prospect of developing new works for a kind of theatre I haven't seen yet though it'll probably incorporate cinema and music in a ritualistic style that's become my signature. I will also keep making films when called by the Muses I follow. I've been given to taking daily walks in the many forests near where I live in Portland, and recommend this ritual to anyone overwhelmed by the static of the default and often toxic culture at large. The trees, they bring me to life.

Antero Alli
Autumn Equinox 2020, Portland OR
http://paratheatrical.com
http://verticalpool.com

orientation

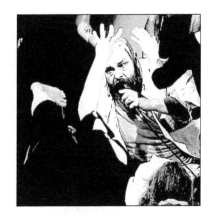

I

PARATHEATRICAL RESEARCH

MIRACULOUS INTERACTIONS OF SELF-GOVERNING BODIES

The phrase "paratheatrical research" came to me in 1977 from the visionary work of the late Polish theatre director, Jerzy Grotowski, whose approaches I deeply respect but am neither emulating nor attempting to replicate. After reading Grotowski's book *Towards a Poor Theatre* and viewing the film document of his Polish Lab's performance of *Akropolis*, I was compelled to continue researching how rituals might work without dogma and how these processes might culminate in a new paratheatrical medium.

One of the ongoing objectives of this medium would be finding methods to discover individual movements, actions and group rituals triggering *miraculous interactions*. They would be miraculous whenever they could invoke (by sound & word) or evoke (by feeling & motion) strong spiritual and visceral resonances erupting in spontaneous gestures, patterns of motion, vocal creations, characterizations and maybe stories that could be shared with others through *resonance*, rather than as linear narratives. Achieving this idea of transmission through resonance would require *an act of total commitment* on behalf of the performer, or ritualist or dancer, to their own spiritual and visceral resonances, resonances that would ripple outwards, like the resonating vibrations of music, to touch others.

Experiencing *the miraculous* requires a kind of double vision capable of holding vertical and horizontal planes together as vertical and horizontal dimensions of existence. The invisible sources of energy and information coming down from above through the crown (top of the head) and the invisible sources of energy and information rising up from below through the soles of the feet and the base of the spine, form a vertical column of energy aligned with the spine. The horizontal plane of energies and information can be experienced as the visible manifestations of our interactions with others, society, political realities, family and the out-there world at large. Vertical is up, down and within; horizontal, out there, around and across. This is no dogma or belief but an attempt at framing this double vision. When individuals choose to interact amongst themselves from a higher commitment to their vertical integrity, conditions are primed for witnessing and engaging the miraculous. When this occurs, a new kind of group unity can develop that doesn't negate the individual but allows for a kind of miraculous interaction of self-governing bodies...

VERTICAL STABILITY

To cultivate resonance with vertical sources is not easy. This kind of inner work persists as an uphill struggle against the grain of decades of horizontal, socially-conditioned, externally-directed habit patterns. Accessing our verticality can act as an irritant to anyone identified exclusively with the horizontal plane of existence. The shock of authentic vertical contact, no matter how fleeting, can shatter unchecked assumptions about the world around us and who we think we are. Any real intimacy with Void (see "The Crux Method of No-Form") can stir deep questioning about identity and the nature of reality.

Some vertically-oriented experiences can act as wake-up calls, alerting us to widespread socio-political oppression in our lives. We may be bolted into outright renunciation and rebellion against all social dogmas, religions and externally imposed belief systems severely compromising our autonomy. However any revolt, no matter how sincere or energized, can prove futile if our very resistance binds us further to the source of our oppression; *we become what we resist*. While breaking out of self-imposed oppressions and our more socially-conditioned habits and reflexes, we must also be willing and able to replace them with a greater force of commitment to our own truths. *It's not what you fight against that matters as much as knowing what is worth fighting for.*

COMMITMENT TO VERTICALITY

When we lose touch with our vertical sources, we lose perspective. Our lives become trivialized in a tangle of meaningless pursuits. We do things without knowing why. We lose track of what is essential to our nature, what matters and what doesn't. All symptoms of power loss. In an attempt to regain lost ground, we may try and assert control by imposing rigid rules and structures over the spontaneous fluidity of life—*our own life or the lives of others*—resulting in a vain and vicious cycle. Loss of vertical context can also result from over-identification with ideas and images lacking vital connection with the realities those concepts supposedly represent; *we eat the menu instead of the meal.* On the other extreme, when we lose our horizontal connection we can suffer loss of community, or common-unity, with our peers. Alienated and isolated, the ego grows brittle, the will to live can wither and we suffer a slow death on the inside or go mad from sheer isolation.

This paratheatrical work is a highly disciplined approach to developing rituals for restoring vertical stability from a fierce stance of personal integrity and autonomy. The degree of commitment required for this approach to work is enormous, commitment to your own direct experience. To work towards this end is challenging; to live your life this way is almost impossible. It can be miraculous.

Instigating a vertical value into any group dynamic often runs against the grain of social expectations. Social gatherings are defined by socially-accepted (horizontal) promises of entertainment, intellectual stimulus, emotional support, ego status, courtship potential and a sense of belonging; all social incentives. When these social motives are replaced by more austere asocial intentions (such as No-Form), they collapse; there's nowhere for them to go.

THE ASOCIAL INTENT

It must be said that this paratheatrical medium works most effectively in *an asocial climate*. Asocial, not to be confused with antisocial, refers to a creative climate where interaction i̶... ba̶sed on meeting social needs. Initiating r̶ meeting in a group starts with realiz- esponsibility to others in the workspace dual vows to be responsible for their own eir own creative states. This pledge mini- ingrained obligations, such as seeking or ance, approval or providing unnecessary protection or acting out courtship behaviors. This self-responsibility frustrates the parent/child fixa- ....ns compelling us to expect others to make us safe and/or to make others feel safe. Taking this vow defines the group as self-accountable adults committed to a crea- tive process, rather than a social one. Anyone unwilling &/or unable to hold themselves to this self-accountability are discouraged to do this work until they are ready to do so.

Becoming responsible for your own safety means tend- ing to your own fears, needs and personal limitations as they emerge. By overlooking these issues it is easy to silently expect others to make you safe, i.e., to be your dad or mum. Making yourself safe prepares the ground for creativity; when a child feels safe, the child can play. Creative states flourish in a state of trust, i.e., feeling safe enough to take risks. The objectives presented in this work depend on your own processes of fulfillment. By finding your own way to realize these goals, you earn more autonomy and integrity.

At first, this adjustment can act as a kind of anxiety-producing social shock or elicit social guilt for indulging in self-centered behavior in groups until assured of their long-term social value. Working in an asocial climate can support new ways of interacting with others from higher levels of individual integrity and autonomy. The goal here is not to develop individuality for its own sake, which merely dead ends in narcissism. Our aim in this paratheatrical work is to discover ways of interacting with others from a deepening sense of personal sovereignty.

Once a paratheatrical group understands from the very start that it is working to cultivate an asocial climate for ritual purposes, a kind of *rare area* can substantiate itself with the second asocial task of *getting your attention off of yourself and onto the space itself.* This literally means relating to the space—the workspace—rather than the things and/or people in that space. How does this occur? By discovering your own way of relating with the space by how you physically move through that space. This task can take anywhere from five to fifteen minutes. (See "Space-Forming" in the next chapter).

NO-FORM: INTIMACY WITH VOID

The void can be pointless to talk, think or write about. Its very nature is not subject to categorization by ideas, images or anything conceptual mind is capable of creating. There are no security, status, symbolic or social rewards given out for being nothing. Nobody wants to be a nobody.

However, as all self-governing bodies eventually realize, real power (not control), real freedom (not ego-independence) and real creativity (not entertainment) stem from any ongoing personal rapport with the formless, invisible sources behind all palpable, visible and manifest effects. To continue interacting with void, we must find ways to refer to it and invite its presence. This state of potential energy is referred to in this medium as No-Form (also see "The Crux Method of No-Form").

THE CONTACT POINT: DIRECT INTUITIVE ENGAGEMENT

From the state of No-Form any quality or force can be accessed through an existing contact point. The contact point is wherever direct, intuitive absorption of a particular energetic state is already happening; one has only to locate it. It already exists in the body as a source of energy. This is an important point to grasp, as the qualities and energies explored in this medium are not always of the imagination. Our biology emanates a complexity of energy dynamics most of which, like the organs themselves, cannot be seen yet each remain vital to the organism as a whole. In fact, these sources of energy are expressions of higher emanations of which our physical organs are also manifestations. *The physical body embodies the so-called Subconscious mind.*

The contact point can also be discovered "non-locally" in the auric field enveloping the physical body and in the space beyond the body's aura, in any area of the setting designated to a particular source. Another way to refer to the contact point is your initial connection with the existing conditions of any quality or source that exists autonomously in its own power and as such, does not have to be imagined or created.

POLARITY WORK

We are complex psychological creatures with opposing forces and contrary realities interacting within our psyches. In this work, we explore the opposing forces of our nature as expressions of a larger changing whole. These inner oppositions are not split but expressions of a great complexity than we may be aware of at the time. Take the polarity of Masculine/Feminine, for example. Masculine energy already exists; we do not need to make it up. From the receptive state of No-Form, we allow its energy to expand from its initial contact point throughout the rest of our body, moving us this way and that, allowing it to infuse our experience with its quality, color and intensity. The energy itself guides the direction rather than our personal will. *Follow the energy, don't push or direct it.*

Polarity work asks us to relax the desire to control or direct the energy. When the force of energy is strong enough to move your body, you follow its direction. By creating space for its expression, you are moved by its force. Like clay in the hands of a sculptor, we are shaped before we start shaping. This takes practice and is nurtured by the authenticity of your No-Form state; the deeper the No-Form, the deeper we can be impressed and moved by a given source through the contact point.

Like the archeologist's pick-axe, this ritual work can be a tool for penetrating the surface crust of social conditioning and mining the veins of our common humanity. To embark on this archeology of the soul, we look to our own personal experiences. This starts with drawing up a polarity list of personally charged polarities made up of strong resistances and/or excitements, of negatively and positively charged personal polarities.

The overall objective of polarity work is to render the emotional ego more flexible. By repeated exposure to opposing sides of one's nature, it becomes more difficult to fixate on any one side over the other. A more malleable ego results, one that can permit more reality. Rendering the ego more flexible completes the physical and emotional cycles of ritual preparation. The body acts as a kind of alchemical alembic, or vessel, containing, mixing, transforming, distilling and refining the constant union of opposites produced by ongoing ritual polarity work. What comes after polarity work depends on the directions suggested by the facilitator or, if the group decides collectively, the mutually agreed upon archetype or theme to explore and the ritual format to best engage those processes.

THE ASOCIAL CLIMATE

THE SOCIAL BYPASS OF
PARATHEATRICAL PROCESS

SPACE-FORMING AND SPATIAL AWARENESS

An asocial climate can be initiated by any action that increases spatial awareness, such as the paratheatrical method of "space-forming." This starts with getting your attention off yourself and redirecting it onto the external space around, below and above you. Once attention can be redirected onto the space itself, you begin moving through that space to discover ways of physically communicating your relationship with the space, moment to moments as you go. As this spatial awareness increases, so does awareness of the personal space around others—the immediate area, or auric field, surrounding each self-governing body. A mutual respect for personal space develops that supports a climate of safety in the group. When we feel more safe, we are more likely to take more risks, such as becoming more vulnerable and available to our internal sources and each other.

A SILENT VOW OF PERSONAL SAFETY

Paratheatrical work can trigger cathartic release, convulsive physical and emotional responses, and sudden loud vocalizations that can throw us and others off balance. In this work, everyone is asked to take a vow to become fully responsible for their own safety and well-being. To be accountable for your own safety means whenever your sense of equilibrium is temporarily interrupted, you simply do your best to restore your sense of safety. *You make yourself safe.* This occurs as a trial-by-error process of experimentation. For example, perhaps you start jumping up and down to feel the soles of your feet to restore your sense of grounding. This vow of personal safety nurtures individual integrity and autonomy, core values in this work. When a group agrees to take this vow, nobody has to wait for anyone else to make them safe. Everyone becomes their own Mom and Dad, so the inner Child can feel safe enough to come out and play.

ASOCIAL INTERPLAY

"Asocial interplay" refers to a paratheatrical process of group interaction that is neither antisocial nor social but a third way of interacting without being socially hostile or socially-conforming. This asocial approach starts with realizing our non-responsibility to others in the workspace. This adjustment initiates a shift from being in a group to meet social needs—*approval, support, affection, acceptance, friendship, courtship, etc. from others*—to being in a group for the work of accessing internal sources and their direct expression through movement, sound, gesture, action. *This shift from the social to the asocial supports greater authenticity of expression and creative response.*

NOT IMPROVISATION BUT AN OFFERING OF SELF

"Asocial interplay" is not the same as improvisation, as commonly defined and known in theatre and dance. In asocial interplay, we want nothing from anybody else nor do we depend on external cues from others (or the audience) to spark or sustain interaction. Asocial interplay sustains itself by each individual's deepening commitment to their own predetermined internal sources. As this internal commitment increases, we apply specific intentions (see "The Five Intentions") to amplify these sources and their expression through vocalization, gesture, action and interaction from higher levels of individual integrity and autonomy. As this self-commitment process deepens, our own presence expands; we have more of ourselves to offer. Asocial interplay supports a spirit of offering of self, rather than a taking or getting from others.

Asocial interaction starts after one's commitment to an internal source reaches its peak and the source energy, or presence, moves one towards a state of offering of the self through spontaneous gesture, action and vocalization. Asocial interplay is never forced, confrontational or encounter-based. In high levels of asocial interplay, we are acted on and influenced by the presence, actions and sounds of others, while our own presence, actions and sounds act on others. Asocial interplay occurs inside this open-ended and unpredictable interaction of self-governing presences. Sustaining concentration amidst this asocial interaction requires a kind of "double vision" that allows total commitment to internal sources while remaining aware of the immediate environment of others.

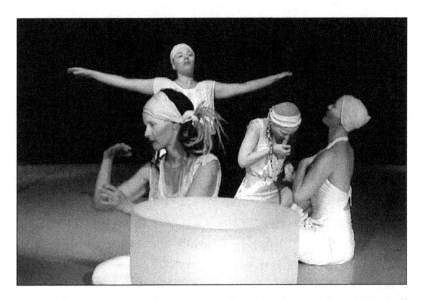

Asocial interplay. The women in the above photo are all sourcing "Divine Feminine" through their own distinctly personal connections. The group unity here does not result from any merging of their energies with each other but from each woman fully committing to her own source while remaining aware of the others and interacting with them from a place of vertical integrity. Self-encounter replaces confronting others.

THE RITUAL FACILITATOR

ON SET AND SETTING, OBSERVATION AND TALKING

This group ritual work has almost always functioned with a Ritual Facilitator as an impartial witness who does not participate in the actual rituals but serves the group as a ritual catalyst. Sometimes, when a given individual becomes adept enough in the work processes, they can join the group on the floor while also acting as Facilitator.

THE SET (MINDSET)

The role of the facilitator is not a director, or a teacher, or a guru, or a therapist. The facilitator is more like a group's "third eye," perceiving the innate dynamics of each session of group work and then, verbalizing simple suggestions for amplifying the existing group dynamics and presenting objectives that each person fulfills in their own way.

THE SETTING (WORKSPACE)

This work process does best under low lighting. Sometimes three of four candles, lanterns, or low wattage bulbs can be enough. About 1000 square feet of open floor space is required for a group of six to twelve (figure 100 sq. ft per person). Wood floors and sprung floors such as those in

dance and yoga studios are best; cement floors can damage ankles and knees when jumping, leaping and jogging.
The workspace should be free of external interruptions
from anyone or anything outside of the group. Unless re-
hearsing for a live performance, any recorded or live music
or percussion can distract from the work of depending on
internal sources for animating expression of sources.
Noise is best kept at a minimum; a quiet setting works
best.

OBSERVING THE EXISTING CONDITIONS

Certain powers of observation are necessary to detect
the present-time moods, needs, resistances and the overall
spirit embodied by any given group during each session.
These observations can begin the moment participants
enter the space and start moving about. The five-phase
physical warm-up cycle is a good time to observe individual and group levels of commitment and energy, or lack
thereof, to see which methods and ritual forms to intro-
duce after the Warm-up—*based on the commitment levels
demonstrated in the warm-up.* The higher the commitment shown in the Warm-up, the more ready the group
may be to engage ritual sources of greater charge, depth
and difficulty. *The more grounded they are, the higher
they can fly.*

DON'T TALK BEFORE OBSERVING

During the work session, participants experience the
facilitator as *a disembodied voice.* Avoid suggestions that
spell things out or define things too much or that require

thinking. Participants want to have an experience, not an explanation. Keep your suggestions simple, direct and somewhat open-ended. Allow space between suggestions; participants need time to discover their own processes. If you're tense, relax. Participants already have enough resistance to deal with without having to also feel yours. The ongoing group dynamics undergo their own changes. At any moment, be ready to adjust your suggestions to the influx of new information. *When in doubt, don't speak.*

TRANSITIONS

The group will sometimes but rarely end each stage of the work session at exactly the same time. After finishing with a source, the group returns to No-Form; some will finish sooner, others later. Pay attention to these transitions between each objective and ritual you suggest. Transitions can tell you what ritual or objective the group might be ready for next or, not ready for. Noting transitions can help you sequence, or layer, the rituals more harmoniously, so each stage of the session supports the next one.

SOURCE WORK

Any source presented in this paratheatrical work is posited as an existing condition, meaning, *as if the source already exists within us.* This approach minimizes cultural concepts and beliefs *about* whatever source is presented while supporting a more direct experience of the source energy itself. Proceeding as if the source already

STATE OF EMERGENCE   39

exists can help stop the mental hijacking of experience
with preconceptions.

CULTIVATING A LACK OF SELF-INVESTMENT

Energetic dynamics are constantly percolating beneath
the threshold of any group and individual consciousness.
The facilitator must know how to perceive these subterra-
nean currents (see the next paragraph, "The First and
Second Attentions"). Start by relaxing "self-investment." If
you are too personally invested in outcomes, participants
will pick up on it and may resist your suggestions. You are
there to support their involvement, not yours. The facilitator acts as a ritual catalyst; *a catalyst doesn't undergo the
same changes as the catalyzed.*

THE FIRST AND SECOND ATTENTIONS

The first attention refers to that awareness linked to
*language, thinking and the assignment of labels and
meanings*; the first attention creates interpretations of
what is perceived. The second attention acts as that awareness linked to *presence, energy and phenomena* without
interpretation or labels. Your words and phrases can better serve the situation when first attention can be trained
to follow the dictates of the intuition of second attention;
let the situation be the boss. Without the second attention,
effective facilitation in this medium may not be possible.

THE FINAL RITUAL OF EACH SESSION

This work activates the energetic body; the sympathetic
function of the Central Nervous System (CNS) becomes

stimulated and "lit." At the end of each session, suggest a final ritual that engages a cooling off process, rather than one that leaves everyone hopped up and wired. Initiating this balance activates the parasympathetic CNS, the rest and restoration function, increasing equilibrium to the more unstable sympathetic CNS. A longer, deeper No-Form helps diffuse the effects of highly charged rituals. *Better to end cool than hot.*

ON THE ENDING GROUP CIRCLE

The sitting group circle that ends each session provides an opportunity to check in, share notes, and voice perceptions. After a particularly charged ritual, participants may be silenced by what happened; don't press them to talk. Those who are ready to talk, will speak. The aim of the group circle is to simply report what happened and provide an opportunity to find language for more in-depth intuitive experiences. If someone starts espousing philosophies and theories about their experiences, gently nudge them back to their actual experience, i.e., *"What happened to you?" "How did you relate to what happened?"* Though philosophical discourse and psychoanalysis have their place, they tend to distance and abstract us from our initial experiences. Be Here Now.

the methods

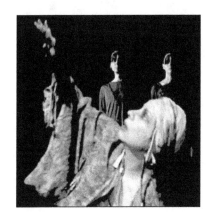

2

THE CRUX METHOD OF NO-FORM

INTIMACY WITH VOID; CREATE TRANCE, BREAK TRANCE

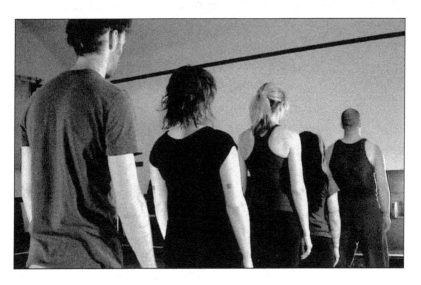

The No-Form experience is approached as a tool to induce enough internal receptivity to engage the vital currents, impulses and autonomous forces innate to the Body *as a movement resource*. In its first function, No-Form acts as a *trance-induction device*. No-Form is implemented after each engagement and expression of energies to discharge and release attachment to these forces. In this way the second function of No-Form acts as *a trance-*

breaking device. No-Form represents the crux method of this paratheatrical work. Not much work of any value can occur until it can be experienced. The following adjustments can support the experience:

THE PHYSICAL STANCE

Stand in any way that supports *vertical rest*—find the point of minimal effort to remain standing, relaxing all muscles uninvolved in this standing posture. *1) unlock the knees 2) widen the stance 3) drop the pelvis 4) let the spine drop and be suspended 5) exhale, allowing the inhale to occur as a reflex and continue this connected breath 6) eyes shut or open a slit to minimize external stimuli.* Notes on breath: By emphasizing the exhale and allowing the inhale to occur as a reflex, the vagus nerve secretes a transmitter substance (ACh) which causes deceleration within the beat-to-beat intervals of the heart via the parasympathetic nervous system (PSNS).

INTERNAL ADJUSTMENTS

Once the physical stance and breath are established: 1) withdraw your attention from the external environment and reconnect internally 2) relax the desire to control the outcome of any experience 3) relax the desire to control 4) find your anchor or comfort at being nothing 5) be nothing.

THE CHARGING ACTION OF NO-FORM

From No-Form, we choose a source to access, say the element of Fire, and posit it as an already existing condition within us. We can project this energy into an area of the workspace, step into that area and allow the Fire element to fill our receptive state. Or we can access Fire right where you are standing. Either way, as the Fire energy begins surfacing within you, don't try to control or direct this energy. Instead, allow the energy to dictate the direction and outcome of your movement, sounds and gestures; let the Fire be the boss. The deeper your receptivity in No-Form, the deeper your experience of whatever source you wish to engage. This initial stage of receptivity and engagement of a source represents the "charging" function of No-Form. *It acts as a trance-induction device if it alters our consciousness from one state to another.*

THE DISCHARGING ACTION OF NO-FORM

Return to No-Form after you're done engaging a source to release your attachment and identification with it. This discharging action of No-Form acts as a trance-dispersion device. By returning to No-Form after each ritual engagement of energies, we intentionally break that trance and restore our receptivity—we return to being nothing or, nobody but ourselves. This return to No-Form minimizes ego inflation that can occur with identification or merging with the psyche's unconscious contents. These two functions of No-Form—*charging and discharging*—occur by setting apart time before and after each ritual immersion to stand in No-Form.

THE FIVE INTENTIONS

DIMENSIONALITY IN SOURCE WORK

The Five Intentions act as devices for opening up *dimensionality* in source work. After the Body is felt deeply during a 25-minute physical warm-up and the group starts approaching a ritual, any of these five intentions can be applied to unlock new dimensions of whatever source is introduced. Sources, such as *The 4 Elements, The Muse archetype, Dreaming, Verticality, and many others,* are all posited as autonomous agencies residing in the Body with lives of their own, often beyond the control and comprehension of the conscious ego. They are assumed to already exist within each of us as psychic realities, as real and sometimes more real than physical realties.

These Five Intentions express a development from the most primitive ("merging") to the most subtle ("inquiry") with each previous intention acting as a support for the following one. Though each intention unlocks a different facet of whatever source is engaged, all five can and do intermingle and influence each other. Each intention represents new ways to engage and express any source. Apply one during any ritual. Come back to them over and over, again, to discover more depth of dimensionality.

1) MERGING (identification)
2) SERVICE (body as vessel)
3) SURRENDER (total offering of self to source)

4) SUSTAINING CARE (finding source empathy)
5) INQUIRY (asking questions of the source)

MERGING (IDENTIFICATION; BECOMING THE SOURCE)

Direct intuitive engagement with the current or energy of any given source, merging represents an *identification* with, and a passive absorbing of whatever the source has to offer. This intention can often erupt in chaotic, convulsive, chaotic and cathartic physical and vocal expressions.

SERVICE (THE BODY AS VESSEL)

After merging with a source, service starts with opening the Body up as a vessel for the source to express *through you*. As the Body becomes as a vessel or medium for the source energy, you are free to not identify or merge with the energy. This freedom expresses an act of *service to the source*, not to ego-identification and satisfaction.

SURRENDER (TOTAL OFFERING OF SELF; FULL EMBODIMENT)

Through merging and service, we can discover enough about a given source to give ourselves over to it towards *a total offering of the self*, the Body, to the source in *a fully embodied expression of the energy*. Surrender differs from the first intention of merging in the way a tree blossoms first before bearing fruit. Surrender expresses the fruition of *total follow-through* of what Merging initiates.

SUSTAINING CARE (WHAT IS LOVED MOST ABOUT SOURCE)

After engaging a source, discover what you love or care most about that source and allow that love and care to sustain your source connection and its expression through you as movement, sound, gesture, action, interaction. The sustaining care intention builds *source empathy* as a sustaining current allowing your entire process to be nurtured by a deepening care and love.

INQUIRY (ASKING QUESTIONS OF THE SOURCE)

Inquiry starts after stepping into a source (from No-Form) and asking that source questions, such as "Where are you going" or "How can I know you?" or "Who are *you?*" Questions should be direct, simple and clear. Questions can also be nonverbal yearnings, such as the quest to discover what you want to know. Inquiry sets up the possibility of dialogue with autonomous sources and can result in the most subtle and sometimes, most profound dimensionality triggered by the five intentions.

TRIGGER METHODS

THE NUTS AND BOLTS OF
THIS RITUAL TECHNOLOGY

In this work the Physical Body is approached *as the living embodiment of the so-called Subconscious*—the internal landscape of impulses, emotion, images, memory, archetypal currents and sensation. In this work, we can gain access to our internal landscapes after meeting the Body's need to be felt deeply (see "The 5-Phase Warm-Up Cycle"). These paratheatrical trigger methods cohere the ritual technology of this medium; apply any one of them during each work session. Returning to them over and over again will expand your ritual skill set and the depths of work you can experience.

INNER ACTIONS

Personal No-Form

The degree of access to the potential state of void marks the starting and ending points for each sourcing ritual. The deeper the capacity for receptivity (via No-Form), the deeper the capacity for experience of whatever energy or source engaged. Personal degree of comfort with being nothing.

Hollow Body

During the No-Form stance, this sense of "hollow body" aims to amplify No-Form; sensing the physical body as hollow, as in, a vessel or a medium.

Impersonal No-Form

Beyond the personal no-form process, Impersonal no-form refers to the potential state beyond one's personal efforts at emptying; the impersonal void at large.

Contact Point

Wherever direct intuitive contact with the energy of a given source already exists—not imagined or visualized but detected as an existing condition. The contact point can appear within the physical body and/or in the energetic body enveloping the physical body, the electromagnetic aura. The degree of detection of the contact point depends on the depth of No-Form.

Conscious Projection

The conscious act of projecting a source of energy into an area on the floor and/or outside of the body and then, physically stepping into that source area to subject yourself to the forces of your own projection. This inner action taps and makes conscious the otherwise unconscious reflex of projecting psychic energy onto others and the world. By making this unconscious process conscious, a ritual technique is born enabling the action of charging an area with a specific energy.

Sourcing

From the receptivity of No-Form, sourcing begins with the inner actions of detecting, accessing, engaging and expressing energy in the body/psyche that leads to full immersion, identification and surrender to direct experience (or gnosis) of that source.

Foundation Source

Executed before the physical warm-up cycle, a single source is chosen and projected onto the entire workspace while standing in No-Form at the periphery of the workspace. From No-Form, you step into the space to engage that source and its expression through you as you navigate the workspace. The foundation source has three purposes: 1) activating the energetic body 2) setting a tone for the following Physical Warm-Up and 3) creating an underlying support source for the entire session.

Active Surrender

When giving oneself over totally to any given source, a state of surrender ensues. Passive surrender internalizes the experience, where outer expression is muted in a kind of caving into oneself. Active surrender allows for a more dynamic outward expression of forces accessed.

Receptive Control

The act of maintaining receptivity to any given source while directing and managing its influence through physical and vocal expression; holding a dynamic balance between spontaneity and precision, control and abandonment.

HUMAN SYSTEMS (INNER & OUTER ACTION COMBINED)

The existing biological systems as sources—*Skeletal, Muscular, Nervous, Respiratory, Circulatory, Glandular, etc.*—as living realities in the Body, rather than as concepts about them. Also used for expanding movement vocabulary beyond pre-existing movement clichés and redundant patterns of motion.

OUTER ACTIONS

Presence Actions

Any action, movement, sound, song or physical adjustment that increases a palpable felt sense of one's own energetic presence and the aura enveloping the physical body. A device for amplifying a direct experience of one's own energy, our "field of presence."

Body as Unit

Moving the body as one unit, as one piece, with no part left behind or isolated from the rest. Much like the way a cat moves across the ground or floor, the cat moves as a unit. Body as Unit incorporates the whole body in motion; like the cat, the movements do not need to be large or dramatic to express unity of the whole body in motion.

Somatic Questions

Three questions are asked of oneself, one at a time allowing for a few minutes each, out loud or in silence: *1) Why am I here? 2) Where am I going? 3) Who am I now?* These questions are asked to invoke somatic response, not any mental conclusions or verbal answers. The Body in motion has its own responses to the questions. Somatic questions aim to liberate the Body's stream of impulses and are often applied before the Physical Warm-up.

Movement Clichés

Consciously exploring redundant movement habits and predictable kinetic patterns towards their full exposure and acceptance. This task identifies those movement styles we tend to repeat and fall back onto as our 'default setting' whenever new movements cease to be discovered.

Movement Vocabulary Work

1) Vertical: any movement limited to up and down directions. 2) Lateral: limited to any sideways movement. 3) Frontal/dorsal: any movement limited to forward and backward motions, tied together as one movement.

Idiosyncratic Motion

The action of allowing whatever state you're in to dictate the expression of movements innate to that state; moving in ways innate to your own energy that cannot be duplicated or copied.

The Movement Stretch

Expanding range of motion by stretching the muscles while remaining in constant movement across the floor. The movement stretch reaches muscles often missed in a stationary stretching process. This action also challenges moment-to-moment awareness while moving across the floor.

Aimless Wandering (wu wei)

Walking about the floor of the space without any intention or any purpose beyond getting lost in a shuffle of aimless wandering. Stopping whenever intention arises and waiting for the impulse of aimlessness to begin.

The Rises

Lying down on the floor and rising to a vertical stance using minimal effort, tension and resistance. The rises help expose any tendency to force or push a movement while increasing awareness of gravity as a propellent for motion and achieving physical verticality with minimal effort. After reaching a vertical stance, fall back to the floor and repeat the process. Rises should be performed at least five times from a different horizontal floor position each time we fall to discover new rising pathways to the vertical stance.

Transitional Jogging

Various jogging forms act as mediums to find or create specific transitions, like a "heat jog" to raise body energy or "maintenance jog" to sustain the heat and presence. Jogging forms also support sourcing and activating the energetic body; "the No-Form jog," "the Verticality jog" and "the non-directional jog."

Follow-Through

The result of allowing any movement, sound, solo or group ritual process to fulfill its natural course to its end; to fully extend any direction towards its natural outcome.

Ritual Actions

Advanced level work—where a given source is expressed through actions and gestures articulating the innate purpose or function of that source.

EMBODIED VOICE WORK

THE UNITY OF SOUND AND MOVEMENT

The Embodied Voice process starts with three steps: 1) sourcing a given energy 2) resonating a sound that matches the frequency of that source and 3) allowing the sound to dictate physical movement. With practice, sound, song and movement blend and unify. The following Embodied Voice methods are best applied to active ritual processes, to singing a song in motion, and/or in physically active toning.

TONING: Resonating a tone on the exhalation; the vibrations of the tone can be moved to different parts of the body, such as, the heart area, the belly or gut, even the legs and the feet.

VERTICAL SOURCE: Two-way column of energy extending down from above the head and through the body and down into the earth below, alongside energy extending up from the earth below, up through the body and up above the head. Accessed in the jog and in the personal space.

IMPULSES: Process of allowing free expression of the body's spontaneous responses to stimulus such as singing your song; unplanned and undirected movements of innate responses to the song.

EARTH: Sourcing the earth's energy as stabilizing current often incorporated in "The Earth Jog" to anchor the attention in the body and resonate sounds and tones that match the frequency of earth energy in the body.

MICRO MOVEMENTS: Very small, sometimes imperceptibly small, movements dictated exclusively by the song's melody.

PRECISION: Clarifying the form and direction of any movement, sound, or song by paring away the excess; any unveiling of the essence of a movement, sound or gesture; finding economy of tone.

SONG ESSENCE: The silent source of the song supporting its own distinct force, quality and tone; with enough commitment to the silent essence of a song, one can find its essential tone.

ESSENTIAL TONE: The tonal essence of the song as discovered through resonating a sound to match the song essence; the essential tone is not the melody of the song but a pre-melodic sound or series of tones.

ANCESTRAL SOURCES: The emotional and spiritual wellsprings of your genetic lineage as represented by a song chosen from the culture of your ancestral legacy; various modes of *song as ancestral vehicle* include: asking them questions, relating to them, singing your song to them, praying to them.

ANCESTRAL RITUAL SONG: The song's core motivation (why the ancestors sang the song you chose. Samples might include: I sing this song for courage to face my losses. I sing this song to stay warm in winter, I sing this song to fight my enemy. I sing this song to honor my elders.

HEAD/HEART/GUT: Technique for singing (or toning) the melody of your song through the three major centers in the body and then, the three minor centers within each. HEAD: throat, mouth, back of head; HEART: lungs, upper chest, upper back; GUT: belly, pelvic basin, solar plexus.

HUMMING: Resonating a tone or melody with the lips together while maintaining space inside the mouth; similar to toning but sound remains in the mouth.

CALL & RESPONSE: Using your song as the only language you have to reach others; requiring moment-to-moment listening and responding.

LAMENT—CELEBRANT: Dynamic song polarity; using your song-as-vehicle to lament and/or celebrate; usually done in groups of three or more.

the rituals

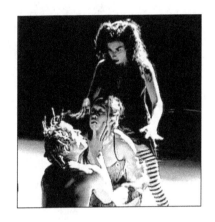

3

THE 5-PHASE WARM-UP CYCLE

TOWARDS FEELING THE BODY DEEPLY

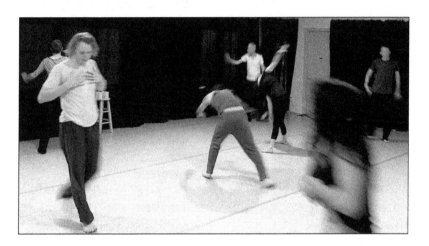

    This PHYSICAL WARM-UP CYCLE initiates every two to three hour work session. Each phase is defined by a specific physical objective: 1) STILLNESS, 2) FLEXING THE SPINE, 3) CORE, 4) STRETCHING, and 5) HEAT. *Everyone in the group meets each objective in their own way.* Each phase runs five minutes. The Ritual Facilitator is responsible for marking five-minute intervals with a bell or a gong. Everyone conducts the entire 5-phase warm-up alone in an area on the floor they have owned and claimed to support a sense of *safety and solitude.* The overall objective of this Warm-Up Cycle *is to feel the body deeply in five ways:*

STILLNESS: any posture supporting physical inaction and meditation to relax the thinking mind.

FLEXING THE SPINE: any process rendering the spine more flexible; this stimulates the nervous systems for more direct passage of signals between the brain and the muscles.

WORKING THE CORE: generating heat and sensation in the abdominal region (yoga, Pilates, crunches, etc.)

STRETCHING THE MUSCLES: breathing into the muscles while stretching; to locate and stretch into "numb" areas.

GENERATING BODY HEAT: any movements, within one's personal area, generating enough heat to break a sweat; raising your physical energy in ways that contain, not disperse, body heat.

Video of the Warm-Up Cycle
http://paratheatrical.com/warmup.html

INITIATION
TO SOURCE WORK

DIRECT ENGAGEMENT &
EXPRESSION OF ENERGIES

The sources introduced in this work, from the Polarities to the Muses archetype, all refer to existing realities rather than any concepts about those realities. The term "sourcing" refers to direct intuitive engagement of a source and its expression through us, through the body, in movement, gesture, action, presence and interaction. Though the aim of all source work is to experience these sources directly, anyone can and probably will encounter preconceptions and ideals about these sources or the cultural and socially-accepted images and models of these realities. For example, when working with the *Masculine* and *Feminine* polarity, stereotypical images and culturally conditioned models of these sources may appear. When these conditioned images surface, let them go or discharge them by openly acting them out until they're rendered ridiculous. Source work can be like peeling layers of an onion to find the heart. *Don't rush. Take your time with every source you engage.*

I view the Body as the living embodiment of the Subconscious. When the Body is felt deeply, as in the 5-phase Warm-up, a kind of door can open to the internal landscape of sources in the Body. If the Body is not felt deeply enough, the door closes and the sources lose power. If you are in the middle of a ritual and become disconnected from your ritual source, your movement loses *organicity*. You may start forcing or pushing the experience, trying to make it happen. When you lose power, don't move; be still. Return to No-Form and restore receptivity. Reboot. Some sources carry more charge, or power, than others depending on their corresponding links within your own psyche. As a rule, the greater the charge of a source, the deeper the No-Form experience may be required to receive that power and also, to discharge that source when you're done.

TRANSITORY JOGGING

Various jogging forms are introduced as transitions between rituals to break the trance of the previous sources and to prepare for the next ritual. These jogs last anywhere from 2 to 5 minutes. Examples of Transitory Jogs include: 1) Heat Jog to raise the physical energy. 2) Maintenance Jog to sustain the heat and presence. 3) No-Form Jog to dissolve any residual identification with sources you're done with. 4) Verticality Jog to restore vertical alignment. 5) Non-directional Jog to relax the grip of tension and control that mentality asserts over the Body. Additional transitory jogs can be created by introducing specific sources while jogging.

POLARITY WORK

THE INTERPLAY OF CONTRARIES

The aim of working with polarities—or contraries—is to increase *ego flexibility* by exposing and releasing previous fixations with one side of any given polarity. This can occur after physically moving back and forth between both sides of the polarity until each side gains equal value. In a group polarity ritual, the workspace is divided in half by an imaginary line separating the chosen polarity. This separating line is designated as a No-Form zone, or a No-Form corridor, where the group stands facing the same direction with the polarity on their left and right sides. With solo polarity work, find and name sources carrying positive and negative charge. *Positive-charge sources genuinely excite you while negative-charge sources carry strong resistance.*

- dreambody/earthbody; masculine/feminine; strong/weak
- order/chaos; nourishing/toxic; dominant/submissive
- stable/volatile; good/evil; commitment/apathy
- safety/danger; mercy/severity; triumph/defeat
- victim/savior; pleasure/pain; precise/sloppy
- dry/moist; repulsion/attraction; known/unknown
- satiated/hungry; mechanical/spontaneous; joy/sorrow
- creation/destruction; illusion/reality; seeing/feeling

- valued/worthless; failure/success; intoxication/sobriety
- heart/heartless; health/illness; love/fear shame/pride
- parent/child; hard/soft; freedom/oppression
- uncertainty/certainty; resistance/non-resistance
- dead/alive; density/clarity; cruelty/empathy
- earth/air; water/fire; lack/abundance
- young/old; beauty/ugly; angles/curves
- red/green; orange/blue; yellow/purple
- head/gut; right/wrong; heaven/hell
- perfect/flawed; silence/noise; creature/spirit
- agony/ecstasy; sacred/profane; control/abandonment
- exposure/shelter; sensitive/numb; acceptance/denial

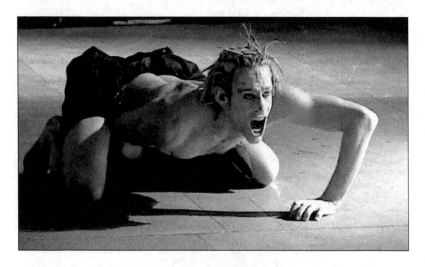

Paradox Pollack from "Orphans of Delirium"
(2004)

THE VERTICALITY RITUAL STRUCTURE

DIFFICULTY LEVEL (I OUT OF 5)

Verticality: the innate stream of energy and information coming down from above through the top of the head, the crown, while simultaneously rising up from below, the earth, up through the soles of our feet and the base of the spinal cord. When this vertical column is experienced directly, the Central Nervous Systems and the energetic body, what Antonin Artaud calls "the double," are activated; we are "lit up" from within. The least difficult ritual in this book (1 out of 5), Verticality is a good place to start group work and can be accomplished in a single three hour session. Or more if you like.

I) SPACE FORMING

The group stands at the outer periphery of the workspace, in a large circle while standing in No-Form, either facing the space or with their backs to the space. After receptivity is established, each person moves into the space—either backwards or forwards—with the intention of discovering ways to relate with the space itself (not the things or people in the space). This is a moment to moment process of physically communicating your relationship with the space as you move through that space.

Include vertical space and the space all around you towards an omnidirectional process of physically relating with the space.

2) FIND YOUR WARM-UP AREA

After exploring the space, find a spot on the floor that somehow resonates or supports your energy. When you find this area, own it. Find movements that express territoriality by claiming this area as yours. Physically demarcate the boundaries and the center of your area. Achieve a sense of being safe and alone.

3) THE PHYSICAL WARM-UP CYCLE

(See "The 5-Phase Warm-Up Cycle")

4) THE VERTICALITY JOG

After the Physical Warm-up, each person starts jogging around the periphery of the workspace towards accessing their Verticality. When this Verticality is established, begin resonating a tone that matches the frequency, the energy, of your Verticality.

5) RETURN TO PERSONAL AREA FOR SOLO VERTICALITY WORK

After the Verticality Jog, return to your warm-up area and reclaim it with the presence of Verticality established in the jog. After this reclaiming, step outside your area and enter No-Form while facing your area. From No-Form, project your Vertical source into your personal area. On reaching peak receptivity, step into your area and surrender to your Verticality. Allow this source to fill you and move you in whatever ways it does. When you feel done or when you exhaust the source, step outside your area and return to No-Form.

6) THE NO-FORM JOG

After your solo Verticality ritual, continue in No-Form by jogging around the periphery of the workspace while sustaining your No-Form process.

7) THE BIO-SYSTEM PASSES

After the No-Form Jog, the group meets on one side of the workspace, shoulder to shoulder, backs to the wall. The entire workspace floor before them is divided into three long rectangular zones (masking or blue tape) designated to the following three bio-systems:

| nervous system |
| muscular system |
| skeletal system |

The group stands in No-Form a few steps from the skeletal system zone. From No-Form, the group steps into the Skeletal system, sourcing and expressing themselves as a skeleton. They move onward into the Muscular system sourcing and expressing themselves as a Muscular system. They move onward into the Nervous system sourcing and expressing themselves as a Nervous system. They move onward into a No-Form zone beyond the Nervous system and discharge the energies. From No-Form, the group returns though the three systems sourcing and expressing themselves as they go until returning to the first No-Form zone past the Skeletal system and discharge the energies.

8) THE VERTICALITY JOG

After the final No-Form of the Group Polarity ritual, start jogging around the periphery of the workspace and return to Verticality. When Verticality is re-established, begin resonating a tone that matches its frequency in your Body.

9) THE GROUP VERTICALITY APPROACH

In the center of the workspace is a circle about 10–15 feet across (marked by tape or candles). This circle is designated to Group Verticality. The group stands at the outer periphery of the workspace in No-Form, facing the space. After No-Form receptivity is established the group approaches the center circle while physically and vocally communicating their relationship with the Vertical source being approached. *Do not rush this approach*; explore this approach itself *as a source*. When ready, enter the center circle and express this Verticality source while remaining aware of others in the circle. When you can sustain Verticality, start opening to others as an offering of presence through gesture, sound and actions. When you feel done or lose power, return to the outer periphery, return to No-Form.

10) THE VERTICAL CHORUS—FINAL RITUAL

The group gathers inside the center circle, facing the center, shoulders barely touching, in No-Form. When receptivity is established, each person begins to resonate tones that match the frequency of the group vertical source. These tones can shift and change, turn into melodies, just so long as you remain committed to the vertical source. When the tones subside, sometimes as if by themselves, the group returns to No-Form. After this final ritual, find a way to break trance and then reconvene for the ending group circle to check in with each other, and share your experiences.

THE FOUR ELEMENTS RITUAL STRUCTURE

DIFFICULTY LEVEL (2 OUT OF 5)

The Four Elements Ritual engages multiple sources—Earth, Water, Fire and Air—as an interrelated, interactive whole. The intent of this ritual is to access all four elements equally towards balancing their energies within oneself. This ritual can be accomplished in a single 3-hour session or repeated over four weeks to gain more depth and substance of experience.

1) FOUNDATION SOURCE

Group stands in No-Form at the outer periphery of the workspace, facing the space. Each person chooses one of the Four Elements and designates the entire workspace to that Element. The element is chosen on the basis on what you need at that moment. Once No-Form receptivity is established, step into the workspace and start sourcing and expressing that Element as you move about.

2) OWNING YOUR PERSONAL AREA

After completing Foundation source, find an area on the floor and claim it with the energy of your chosen element. Physically demarcate the boundaries and the center of your area. Achieve a sense of safety and solitude here.

3) PHYSICAL WARM-UP

(See "The 5-Phase Warm-up Cycle"). Stay connected with your chosen elect through all five phases of the Warm-Up cycle.

4) THE VERTICAL CONTAINMENT JOG

After the Warm-Up cycle, jog around the periphery of the workspace in such a way as to contain the heat and presence you generated in the Warm-Up. Once contained, begin sourcing Verticality as a contained process; The Vertical Containment Jog.

5) ELEMENTAL GROUP POLARITY

Divide the workspace in half with the dividing line designated as a No-Form corridor where the group stands single file in No-Form. Designate the left side of the space to your chosen Element and the right side of the space to the opposite element. Earth/Air and Water/Fire are natural opposites. In No-Form, enter the side that exerts the greater "pull." Visit each side of this elemental polarity at least twice before returning to the No-Form corridor to discharge the energies you've absorbed and expressed.

6) THE NON-DIRECTIONAL JOG

After the Group Element Polarity, jog around the periphery of the workspace while relaxing the grip over your body to achieve a kind of rag doll looseness, letting go of any residual sourcing energies. This is a jog of "controlled

abandonment," sustaining just enough self-awareness not
to fall, bump into others, or injure yourself.

7) THE FOUR ELEMENTS, PT. I

NOTE: A large area, 20–30 feet across the workspace
floor, has either been previously drawn and quartered with
masking tape or demarcated with four candles to create
the boundaries of four separate contained areas within a
large circle. The quadrants are designate to AIR, to FIRE,
to EARTH and to WATER. (see below)

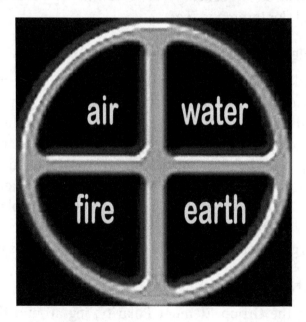

Everyone stands in No-Form a foot or so outside the
large circle, facing the center. From No-Form, each person
enters the closest quadrant to where they are standing and
starts sourcing that element, finding its expression as
movement, sound, patterns of motion, and gestures

organic to that element. When this experience has fulfilled itself, each person moves to another quadrant repeating this process until all four elements have been experienced and expressed by each person. At that time, each person returns to No-Form outside the circle.

8) THE FOUR ELEMENTS PT. 2 (CHOOSE AN ELEMENT)

Outside of circle, each person chooses the element they either feel the greatest need for or that was the weakest element. From No-Form, enter the chosen quadrant to deepen the experience and expression of the element there. While staying connected to that element, start navigating around the other three quadrants. For example, if you start with Fire, you stay with Fire as you pass through Water, Air and Earth. Staying true to your source element, be open to interacting with others *through the expression of your element.* If you disconnect with your element and lose power, return to your element quadrant and replenish your source there. And then, return to the other elements, staying true to your source while interacting with others. When each person feels done, they return to the periphery for No-Form.

9) RETURN TO NON-DIRECTIONAL JOG

After the Four Elements Group ritual, everyone jogs around the periphery of the workspace finding the rag doll looseness allowing the release of any residual elemental energies.

10) THE ELEMENTAL CHORUS/GROUP CIRCLE

After the Non-directional Jog (3–5 min.), the group returns to the Elemental circle, standing in a tight No-Form circle facing the center, shoulders barely touching. Whatever quadrant/element each person is standing in becomes the source they are drawing from for this final ritual. From No-Form each person absorbs the element they are standing in and resonates a tone that matches the frequency of that element. Allow the sounds and tones to undergo their own changes and harmonics. After the Elemental Chorus fades out on its own, the group sits down right where they are to check in, share notes, voice their experiences.

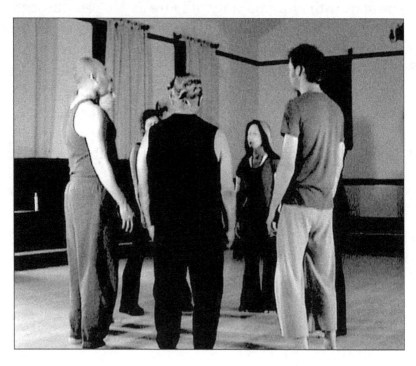

THE DREAMING RITUAL STRUCTURE

DIFFICULTY LEVEL (3 OUT OF 5)

The mid-range difficulty (3 out of 5) of this Dreaming Ritual may start with the attempt to recall *movements* from dreams, a different kind of memory than remembering faces or colors or places in dreams. These movements don't have to belong exclusively to your dreambody, but can be from other dream entities, human, animal or otherwise. They also don't have to be from the same dream as long as they originate in the dreamtime. You must be able to physically replicate each movement on awakening and perform it as close to how it was recalled in the dream. This ritual requires *no less than three movements and no more than five* to build your dreaming ritual choreography.

NOTE: Due to the challenge of recalling dream movements, this ritual has required more time than the other four rituals in this book. Some groups met for three or four sessions before everyone found their dream movements. This ritual has done well in a 4 to 6 week Lab schedule, meeting once or twice a week for 3 hours each time.

1) FOUNDATION SOURCE: DREAMBODY

Group stands at the outer periphery of the workspace in No-Form, facing the space. Everyone designates the entire workspace to Dreambody as a source. Once receptivity is established, enter the space and start sourcing, embodying and expressing the Dreambody as you go. Find your Dreambody movement style.

2) FIND YOUR WARM-UP AREA

After the Foundation source, find a spot on the floor for the warm-up cycle and own it with the Dreambody source. Physically demarcate the boundaries and the center of your area. Achieve a sense of being safe and alone here.

3) THE PHYSICAL WARM-UP CYCLE

(See "The 5-Phase Warm-up Cycle").

4) GROUP POLARITY: DREAMBODY/EARTHBODY

Directly after the Warm-up, the group files into the No-Form corridor dividing the workspace in half for the dreambody/earthbody Group Polarity. Designate the left side to *the dreambody* and the right side to *the earthbody* (your daytime mundane self). From No-Form, enter whichever side exerts the greater "pull." Visit each side of this dreambody/earthbody polarity three times before returning to the No-Form corridor to discharge the energies you've absorbed and expressed.

5) THE EARTH JOG

After the Group Polarity, jog around the periphery of the workspace sourcing the energy of the earth below through the soles of your feet and the base of your spine. Allow the power of the earth to influence your jog. When this energy has stabilized, begin resonating a tone that matches the frequency of the earth energy as you jog.

6) THE NO-FORM-DREAM-FORM CONTINUUM

After the Earth Jog, the group meets on one side of the workspace, shoulder to shoulder, backs to the wall in No-Form. The entire workspace floor before them is divided into three long rectangular zones (marked with masking taped and/or candles) designated to the following three zones:

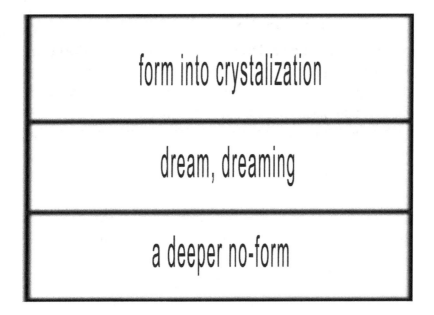

form into crystalization

dream, dreaming

a deeper no-form

The group stands in No-Form a few steps from the "deeper no-form" zone and steps into it absorbing a greater depth of No-Form. Then you step into the "dream zone" sourcing and expressing the dreaming. In the "dream zone," follow any pathway into the "form zone" and crystallize this direction into an extreme full body gesture; hold still for ten seconds. Then move beyond the "form zone" into No-Form (beyond "Form") to release the crystallized form. From No-Form, return to the "form zone" and inhabit the previous crystalized form for ten seconds. Then, enter the dream zone and onward into the "deepening no-form zone" before arriving at the personal No-Form spot where the passes started. This full pass (there and back) through the No-Form-Dream-Form continuum needs repeating one more time.

7) THE DREAM MOVEMENT CYCLE (15–20 MINUTES)

After the No-Form/Dream/Form continuum, the group is ready to start building and practicing their dream ritual choreography, the final preparation for the Dreaming Ritual. The sequence of your dream movements doesn't matter. What matters is how well they all flow together as one fluid movement cycle.

Decide which movement will be the first one. Link the end of the first movement to the beginning of the second movement to form a longer movement combining the two. Practice this two-part movement for a few minutes until it becomes one fluid motion of two parts. Then, link the end of the second movement to the beginning of the third to create a new movement combining all three together. Practice this 3-part combination until it becomes fluid and your body has memorized it. Finally, connect the end of the third motion to the start of the first one. Practice this movement cycle until it flows and your body memorizes it. (If you have four or five movements, extend the cycle to include them; more than five movements over-complicates this ritual). Practice the entire movement cycle until it becomes a fluid dance with its own rhythms. Let any dream memories, images or feelings surface but stay committed to maintaining the integrity of the movement cycle. Practice this cycle for five to ten minutes or until you don't have to think about it; do it until it becomes second nature.

8) THE HEAT JOG

After creating the physical part of the dream choreography, the group jogs around the periphery of the room in any way that generates body heat and energy in a Heat Jog. The dual aim of this Heat Jog is to break the trance of creating the choreography and raising enough energy to animate the Dreaming Ritual.

9) THE DREAMING RITUAL

The group stands at the outer periphery of the workspace in No-Form, facing the space. Designate the entire workspace to the *presence and power of the dreaming*. Remain in No-Form while sensing the area before you and its presence of the dreaming. From No-Form, enter the charged "dreaming" space and stand there and be still, absorbing the power of dreaming. Let this power fill you and move you in whatever ways it does. Do not try and control or direct this energy; let it direct and guide you. When you feel full with the dreaming, begin practicing your movement cycle.

NOTE: The pace, form or rhythm of your movement cycle may shift or warp due to the influx of the "dream charge." Work to maintain the structural integrity of the movements while being guided by the power of dreaming.

As you continue the movement cycle, allow any images and emotions to flow up and influence your ritual. Do your best to stay true to your dream choreography. If you lose structural integrity (when your choreography falls apart) or when you lose power (the dreaming force disappears), return to the periphery of the space and return to No-Form. Start the dreaming ritual over.

Continue executing your ritual choreography under the influence of the dreaming zone until you feel done or when your choreography falls apart or when you lose power if the dreaming force disappears.

10) CLOSURE

Return to No-Form at the periphery of the workspace. Release any attachment to the dreaming power and send it back to its source. When you feel empty, jog around the periphery of the workspace for about a minute to break trance and then meet the others in the ending group circle to check in and share experiences.

NOTE: *dreambody/earthbody,* a video document on this dreaming ritual can be watched at:

http://paratheatrical.com/dreambody.html

SAVIOR, VICTIM, PERSECUTOR RITUAL (SHADOW WORK)

DIFFICULTY LEVEL (4 OUT OF 5)

The difficulty level of this Savior/Persecutor/Victim ritual (4 out of 5) can be defined by the Shadow work it represents. All three archetypes of this trinity can carry different levels of charge, or power, depending on the degree any have been repressed and/or denied within oneself. This difficulty can be supported with a committed physical warm-up, a personal polarity, more depth of No-Form, and enough honesty and self-compassion to face more truth about yourself.

NOTE: This ritual requires research beyond the workspace to identify a personal polarity of sources carrying strong positive and negative charge. Positive-charged sources will excite you; negative-charged sources elicit strong resistance. Examples: *failure/success, triumph/ defeat, control/abandonment* (also see "Polarity Work").

1) SOMATIC QUESTIONS (7–10 MIN.)

Three questions are asked of oneself, one at a time, allowing for a few minutes each, spoken out loud or in silence: *1) Why am I here? 2) Where am I going? 3) Who am I now?* These questions are asked for somatic response, not for mental conclusions or verbal answers. Speak to the Body. The Body will have its own responses to each question when repeated. Somatic questions aim to liberate the Body's stream of impulses.

2) OWN YOUR WARM-UP AREA (WITH THIRD QUESTION)

Follow the Body's responses to the final question "Who am I now?" to your warm-up area and claim it with your somatic responses to this question. Physically demarcate the boundaries and the center. Achieve a sense of being safe and alone.

3) THE PHYSICAL WARM-UP CYCLE

(See "The 5-Phase Warm-up Cycle")

4) PERSONAL POLARITY WORK

Directly after the warm-up, step outside of your area, into No-Form while facing the area. Mentally divide your area into two halves, assigning each side to the sources of your chosen polarity. Best to use a polarity of sources carrying strong positive and negative charge. *Positive-charged sources will excite you; negative-charged sources elicit strong resistance.* Enter your area, exploring one side and then, move to the other side; go back and forth and visit both sides at least twice. *Return to No-Form.*

5) THE NO-FORM JOG

After the Personal Polarity in No-Form, start jogging around the periphery of the workspace while sustaining your No-Form process.

6) THE MOTHER/CHILD/FATHER PASSES

After the No-Form jog, the group meets on one side of the workspace, backs to the wall, facing the workspace. The workspace floor is divided into three long rectangular zones (with masking tape and/or candles) designated to these three archetypes:

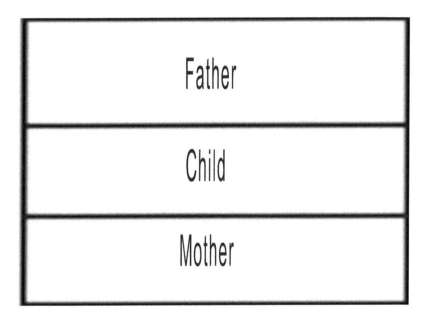

The group stands in No-Form a few steps in front of the Mother zone. From No-Form, the group steps into Mother, sourcing and expressing themselves. They move onward into sourcing the Child. They move onward into sourcing the Father. Then they move beyond Father into a No-Form zone to discharge the energies. From No-Form, the group returns through the three zones while also *sourcing the transitions between them.*

NOTE: This trinity includes all correlations to Mother, Child, Father: *our gene pool to family conditioning (upbringing) to the universal archetypes of this trinity.* When everyone reaches final No-Form, they then jog around the workspace.

7) THE VERTICALITY JOG

Jog around workspace periphery sourcing Verticality while resonating a tone that matches the frequency, the energy, of your Vertical source.

8) SAVIOR/VICTIM/PERSECUTOR PASSES

After the Verticality Jog, the group meets on same side of the workspace as the previous Passes, backs to the wall, facing the workspace. The workspace floor is divided into three long rectangular zones (masking tape or candles) designated to:

```
┌─────────────────────────────────┐
│                                 │
│          Persecutor             │
│                                 │
├─────────────────────────────────┤
│                                 │
│            Victim               │
│                                 │
├─────────────────────────────────┤
│                                 │
│            Savior               │
│                                 │
└─────────────────────────────────┘
```

The group stands in No-Form a few steps in front of the Savior zone. From No-Form, the group steps into Savior, sourcing and expressing themselves. They move onward to source the Victim. They move onward into sourcing the Persecutor. Then they move beyond Persecutor into a No-Form zone to discharge the energies. From No-Form, the group returns back though the three zones, from Persecutor into Victim into Savior and back to No-Form past the Savior.

9) THE HEAT JOG

After the previous Savior, Victim, Persecutor passes, the group jogs around the workspace periphery in any way that raises their physical energy in a Heat Jog to meet the demands of the following Temple ritual.

10) THE SAVIOR/VICTIM/PERSECUTOR TEMPLE

The workspace floor is framed by a large equilateral triangle with three candles or lanterns placed as altars, designated to each of the three archetypes. Let these altars represent portals of each archetype. Designate the lines connecting all the altars as *pathways between the archetypes*, pathways that also act as sources unto themselves.

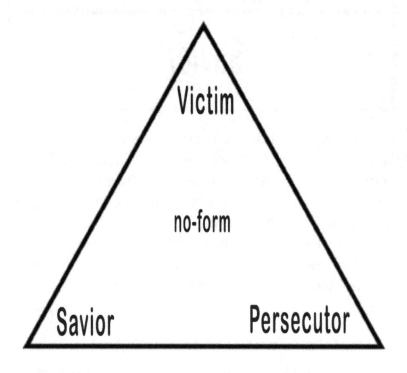

RITUAL INTENT

The group stands in a No-Form circle, shoulder to shoulder, facing outwards, at the center of the triangle. From No-Form, each person steps forward to engage their closest pathway or altar source. The aim here is to navigate the Temple along the pathways—*as approaches and departures from each altar archetype*—and, to surrender to each archetype when arriving at its altar. Any time you lose power or become disconnected from any source, return to the center No-Form circle and start over. It doesn't matter if you navigate the pathways clockwise or counter-clockwise, as long you commit to the pathway as a source that either approaches an altar archetype or departs from an altar archetype. Pathway sourcing is about expressing the approach and the departure from an archetype. Ritual ends with a return to No-Form at the center.

11) THE NO-FORM JOG

After the Temple ritual, begin jogging around the periphery of the workspace while sustaining your No-Form process.

12) IMPERSONAL NO-FORM (FINAL COOLING OFF)

The group stands at the outer periphery of the work-space in No-Form while facing the space that is designated to IMPERSONAL NO-FORM. Beyond the personal No-Form experience, *Impersonal No-form* refers to the potential state outside of one's personal efforts and processes, the impersonal void beckons from the beyond.

After personal No-Form receptivity is established, step into the Impersonal No-Form area and let yourself be *acted on by its all-pervasive impersonal presence*. When you're done navigating Impersonal No-Form, return to the workspace periphery and enter your personal No-Form process (note the difference between the personal and impersonal No-Form). The group convenes in a seated group circle to check in and share experiences.

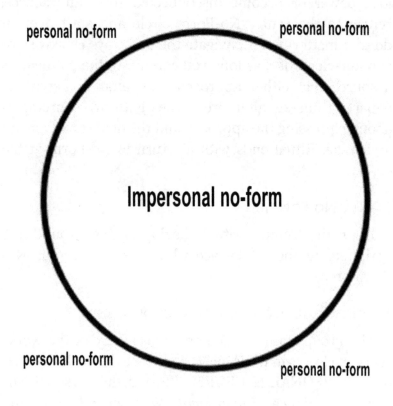

THE MUSES RITUAL STRUCTURE

DIFFICULTY LEVEL (5 OUT OF 5)

The most difficult ritual in this book (5 of 5) requires an already existing resonance or a feeling for archetypal experience as a source of inspiration. Add to this more depth of No-Form practice, a very high commitment in the warm-up cycle and insight into choosing a personal holy trinity (see next paragraph). The MUSES ritual explores keys for unlocking the Muses archetype—not *"my Muse"* or *"your Muse" (they belong to no one!)* **but the Muses.** In this ritual, The Muses are approached as an autonomous, numinous archetype, singular and/or plural, functioning independent of ego (this Muses ritual was explored over seven separate paratheatrical Labs between 2010 and 2019, meeting once or twice a week for three hours over 5–10 weeks).

THE HOLY TRINITY: This ritual requires research beyond the workspace to identify a *personal holy trinity* of sources representing the three most essential sources of your life, as you know it. If they are truly essential, you are not willing to live without them. For example, one of my holy trinities is Love, Ritual and Music. Everyone in the group must arrive at this Muses ritual with their holy trinity.

1) THE RISES

Objective: Lying down on the floor, start rising to a vertical stance using minimal effort, tension and resistance. The rises expose any tendency to force or push a movement while increasing awareness of gravity as a propellent for motion and achieving physical verticality with minimal effort. After reaching a vertical stance, fall back to the floor and repeat the process at least five times from a different horizontal floor position each time to discover new rising pathways to the vertical stance.

2) FIND YOUR WARM-UP AREA

While navigating the Impersonal Void, settle on a spot on the floor and start claiming this area for your warm-up. Physically demarcate the boundaries and the center of your area. Achieve a sense of being safe and alone here.

3) THE PHYSICAL WARM-UP

(See "The 5-Phase Warm-up Cycle"). You are warming up for your Holy Trinity.

After the heat cycle of the Warm-Up, step outside your area facing it. Start your own personal process of No-Form. Divide your personal area into thirds for the three sources of your trinity and step inside your area and, one at a time, explore all three sources. Visit each one two or three times.

4) THE NONDIRECTIONAL JOG

After the solo Holy Trinity work, jog around the periphery of the workspace while relaxing any mental grip you feel over the physical body, releasing excess tensions towards a kind of rag doll looseness. Find your point of controlled abandonment by letting go of enough control without falling or hurting anyone.

5) HEAD/HEART/GUT PASSES

After the NonDirectional jog, the group meets on one side of the workspace, backs to the wall, facing the workspace. The workspace floor is divided into three long rectangular zones (with masking tape and/or candles) designated to three centers in the Body:

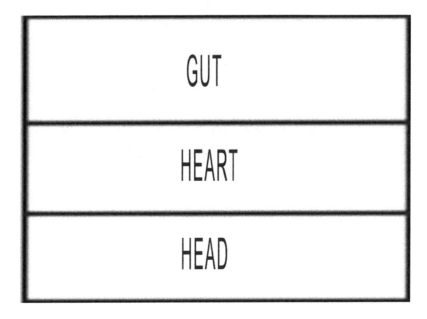

This trinity refers to the existing conditions of energy in one's head, heart and gut. Take your time with this trinity and vocalize these sources as you move (see "Embodied Voice Work"). The group stands in No-Form a few steps from the Head zone. From No-Form, step into Head, sourcing and expressing this energy. Then onward to sourcing Heart. Then onward into sourcing the Gut. Then, move to a No-Form zone beyond Gut to discharge these energies. From No-Form, return through all three zones while also *sourcing the transitions between them.* Return to No-Form.

6) THE HEAT JOG

After the Head/Heart/Gut passes, jog around the workspace periphery to raise your physical energy in a Heat Jog for meeting the demands of the Muses ritual.

7) THE MUSES RITUAL, PT. I DRESSING THE TEMPLE

After the Heat Jog, the group meets on same side of the workspace as the previous Passes, backs to the wall, facing the workspace. The workspace floor is divided into two areas (masking tape or candles), one larger than the other and designated to:

```
┌─────────────────────────────────────────┐
│                                           │
│         Temple of the Muses               │
│                                           │
├───────────────────────────────────────────┤
│                                           │
│                                           │
│                                           │
│         The Holy Trinity Realm            │
│                                           │
│                                           │
│                                           │
└─────────────────────────────────────────┘
```

The Muses Temple is designated as the residence or portal of the Muses archetype. The Muses Temple need dressing with numerous candles and draped fabric to set it apart aesthetically from the Holy Trinity realm which remains empty and dark. The Holy Trinity realm provides a space for sourcing one's trinity, finding your trinity dance before approaching the Muses and a place to restore your trinity sources if they lose power (described below).

(The Muse Temple should be dressed before the session starts.)

PART I: Sourcing the Trinity, Approaching the Muses

The group, in No-Form, faces the Holy Trinity realm and Muses Temple beyond it. Stepping into Holy Trinity realm, access one of three sources of your trinity. After that first source, move onto the second source and then, the third source. Shift between all three sources until they start blending together; stay aware of the Muses Temple. Once blended, enter the Muses Temple and *let the archetype act on you.*

While in the Muses Temple continue expressing—*in gesture, movement and sound*—how the Muses archetype is *acting on you.* Take your time. Remain in the Muses Temple until called back to the Holy Trinity realm, either from Muses overwhelm and/or the need to renew your internal trinity.

8) THE MUSES RITUAL, PT. 2 DANCING INTO THE MUSES TEMPLE

After completing Part 1, either from exhaustion or source disconnect or just feeling done with that cycle, return to No-Form and stand facing the Holy Trinity realm and the Muses Temple beyond.

From No-Form, step into the Holy Trinity realm, and access one of your three trinity sources with the intention of finding a movement that's organic to that source alone. Then, move onto the second source and find a movement organic to that source. And finally, do the same with the third source of our trinity. Begin combining all three movements together (much like the "The Dreaming Ritual" movements) into a dance. Practice this ritual trinity dance until it becomes fluid and pleasurable.

When you're ready, dance into the Muses Temple and allow the Muses archetype to act on you and your trinity dance. Take your time. Remain in the Muses Temple until called back to the Holy Trinity realm, either from Muses overwhelm and/or the need to renew your internal trinity. At this point, you can return to No-Form beyond the Holy Trinity realm or dance back into the Muses Temple; your call. When the group is done, return to No-Form outside of the Holy Trinity realm.

9) THE NO-FORM JOG

After the Muses ritual, start jogging around the periphery of the workspace while sustaining your No-Form process. After the jog, convene in a group circle on the floor to check in and share your experiences.

lab reports

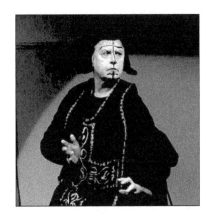

4

PARTICIPANT EXPERIENCES

REPORTS FROM THOSE WHO HAVE DONE THIS WORK

The following stories are from individuals who have undergone this paratheatrical training from the short term (two or three 8-week Labs) to the long term (10 years and more).

NICK WALKER, Aikido Sensei

I was a regular participant in the work of Paratheatrical Research between 1999 and 2015. Long-term engagement with this work has been, and continues to be, an ongoing process of growth and transformation; a process of opening to, and integrating, the new and the long-lost, the hidden and the liminal, Self and Shadow, the archetypal and the transcendent.

In the Paratheatrical labs, on the wooden floor with the other lab participants, I do the work of opening to these forces, these energies, these intelligences and potentials. I invite them to dance with me, or maybe they invite me to dance with them. I get to know them by allowing them to move me.

But that's only where the work begins. The greater part of the work happens outside of the Paratheatre lab space, out in the rest of my life, as I integrate my lab experiences. Because each force with which I dance in the lab space poses a challenge to me: "Can you make room for me in your life? Can you make room for me in your in your psyche, in your everyday self-embodiment and self-concept, in your practice, in your creative work, in the ways you dance with others and with the world?"

A bold new gesture emerges in one of my dances in lab, and demands, "Can you make a gesture this big and bold when you're teaching in the college classroom?"

A deep song emerges from my belly in lab, and demands, "Can you speak from this depth in your next public speaking engagement?"

A new rhythm emerges in my body in lab, drummed out on the floor with my hands and feet, and it lingers in my body and demands that I acquire a big drum, put it in my living room, and take up a daily drumming practice.

A profound spirit of love envelops me and moves me in lab, and demands, "Can you embody this in your aikido practice? Can you transmit it to your aikido students?"

Waves of ecstatic laughter rush through me in lab, pour from me, rock my body, and demand, "Can you dare to be a Fool now and again in your life, dare to surrender to impulse, to wonder, to laughter, to spontaneous urges to dance, to sudden attacks of poetry?"

SYLVI ALLI, Singer/Musician

2010. For the past ten years I have participated in Antero Alli's paratheatre ritual labs fairly consistently, and this work has had a profound impact upon my life. I acknowledge that I will never be able to communicate with words the places and miraculous encounters my psyche has traversed in the course of this work, but I will share some of the ways that participating in paratheatre has initiated change in me.

Starting with my most recent immersion in the ritual work—The Alchemy Lab—I am emerging from this 3-month lab with a stronger grasp of "process," the continuing journey, replete with cycles: tending the seed, fruition, death, rebirth...the open-ended process of my own individual life. I have also become increasingly aware of the value of and my need for receptivity, in all aspects of my life—especially creative, relational, spiritual—and how this receptive state demands true stillness, as well as deeper listening.

Overall, the paratheatre work has had an effect of breaking down my self-imposed boundaries, limitations and fixed ideas. And this, in turn, has strongly affected the degree of self-consciousness that I move through life with. When I first began this work, my self-consciousness level was extremely high, but over the years, as my commitment to the work has deepened, I have experienced a lessening and, at times, a complete absence of self-consciousness. I have gained more freedom, especially in the area of expression—expression of energies, expression of self.

Another way this work has strongly influenced my life is in the area of "not knowing." Where, at one time, I viewed "not knowing" as a huge problem, now this state of uncertainty, of not having a preconception of what lies ahead, has proven to be the very realm of magic, of creativity, of miracles, even... Everything I've mentioned here is tied in to what is at the crux of this work, letting go, emptying out—the practice of No Form—No Form Rules!

JULIAN SIMEON

I first met Antero about 30 years ago. I was a graduate student in an innovative wilderness psychology program at Sonoma State University. I was working towards a minor in Theatre and was taking a mime class with solo stage actor, Fred Curchack. Antero substituted a few of the classes in Fred's absence. My body can still remember the first exercise this "X-Factor sub" had the class attempt. Our task was to find a "way" to move across the room and end the movement in a tableau. We did it over and over again. It was like wind sprints for aspiring ritual actors. I loved it.

As part of rehearsals Antero introduced a working modality he called Ritual Theatre (RT). I fondly recall that wilderness Professor Robert Greenway gave Antero a key to Steven's Hall so our RT group could access classroom space to work...sometimes starting at midnight. The intrigue of his work caught more than my attention. As a participant in the RT work I was able to access fleeting moments and insights that I had only experienced through work with entheogens or out on a long wilderness trip. This drug free modality had me hooked. Hmmm... I thought. I like this work.

Working with Antero over the years, I have been in a few live ritual theatre performances, three or four video films, and numerous RT labs. I take breaks from the Work from time to time. Some longer than others. But when my Spirit yearns to worship and pray, then it is time for me to seek the next lab. Ritual Theatre is a vehicle which when worked at with intent and commitment can take one to places not accessible under "normal" conditions. I thank Antero Alli for his dedication to the Work. His Work. I am grateful to have met him and call him Friend.

HELIA RASTI, Naturopathic Doctor/Acupuncturist

My initial pull to paratheatre came from a desire to understand how theatre could be used to facilitate healing transformation. This stemmed from a practical curiosity as a student/practitioner of acupuncture, and also from a personal yearning to grow as an artist by engaging in creative work. I was elated to find that the practice is one of radical freedom and cathartic release. I was invited to explore the sources of my obsessions, of my dreams, and of my life's purpose—in short, to explore the very essence of my being.

Connecting to no-form and deepening my surrender to these sources allowed me to unwind and release entrenched psychic patterns, by bringing them into physical form. I learned to connect more fully with my heart, and to deepen my sense of intuition.

I'm deeply grateful for the experience and continue to draw from it in my clinical practice, which requires me to identify subtleties in Qi dynamic in order to achieve correct diagnosis and treatment.

JAMES WAGNER, Actor

My driving intention is to actualize my gift as an actor as a full spectrum spiritual practice. I came to paratheatre to explore and develop that possibility. I can say that without question, my experiences in paratheatre have been the single greatest tool I've found to meet my intention. It has revolutionized my being and thus revolutionized my art.

For me, surrender, submission and service to autonomous energy sources in a full committed and active physical/vocal expression (and the personal preparatory work necessary to make my body capable of that service) is the core value I receive from the work. I now approach my entire artistic process as excavation, submission, surrender and service founded on as much spaciousness and receptivity as possible (which comes through deepening practice of no-form). I also have been able to significantly deflate (and "right-size") the role of my ego in the process. I now often languish in the joy that accompanies the Real Experience of a Divine Force in its many manifestations as the source and guide of all creative (and life) processes. Connection to and Knowledge of That Force and submission to its will through art (giving it form through creative action) is a great gift and a great relief.

That said, the fire of self-exposure has been excruciating and of course, eventually, relieving and liberating. I bow in gratitude to Impersonal No-Form that secretly animates this whole endeavor.

TREY DONOVAN, Dancer/Musician

I appreciated the methodical approach of a timed warmup, so that there was not any guesswork about where to focus energy at this specific part of the work, and yet enough latitude to determine my own method in each of the phases of physical warmup. The prescribed rituals I felt were quite simple to grasp as were relationships between source, for example, the division of the room into named quadrants that touched one another in, at once, a conceptual and a profound way provided a framework that I readily could apply what I already know, yet could immerse fully into as mystery, as well.

What I didn't expect and what visited me pretty much in each of the 7 lab sessions was a visit from the work I've done in Subud. Something tells me that opening oneself up to vertical sources induces the soul body to connect with a timeless part of one's life. At least that is my considered opinion, based on what was happening, seemingly involuntarily, when participating in the lab. Seems to me that what is being approached in the paratheater work is preparation for real spiritual work. This is something that I feel has been impossible for me to do while sitting in silent meditation, but in Paratheater, appears to open up.

My particular manifestation of this is very distinct and I recognize it instantly. So when that crept up, I was not surprised, but I didn't expect it. Things that appeared to me as answers to burning spiritual questions out of this Paratheater work were also occasionally unexpected, but welcome. I was very happy to get some of these answers, and others of these answers have been kind of vexing and disturbing. But the truth is not always what we want to see...so to honor my own truth is probably my biggest take-away from the Basics lab.

JESSICA BOCKLER, Ph.D., Performer/Teacher

Just over a year ago I followed a hunch. Whilst researching Jerzy Grotowski's work on the internet I came across Antero Alli's website and work. I was immediately fascinated... Everything I read on the site was so much what I was striving for as a theatre practitioner, artist and writer... Everything I read was so much about what I needed as a human being. And so I set my intention...to travel from Liverpool in the UK to Berkeley...to participate in Antero's Alchemy Laboratory in the spring of 2006.

What I encountered in this lab is something I will never forget—yet it is still largely ineffable. The work was intense, powerful, demanding, exploratory yet disciplined, tedious yet exhilarating, carefully structured yet utterly unpredictable. I loved almost every moment of it...and I now deeply appreciate the moments of frustration, fear and disorientation I experienced when things didn't go so smoothly for me! Indeed, those moments were an essential part of the journey...they helped me gain a deeper insight into myself...and I feel that I have grown as an artist and as a person. Antero, thank you so much for the adventurous ride! I hope I may find my way back to you in the coming years!

ISHMAEL AYLWIN

Paratheatre work pushed me to explore my nervous system somatically and then discover what I knew, but had no conscious awareness of. The practice endeavored to break my conscious habitual neural net patterns of thought by taking me directly to my body and asking me to change somatic holding patterns there, especially as expressed through movement. Since my mind and body are two sides of one coin, this process forced me to change how I thought as well as how I moved. The challenge was to remain receptive enough to allow conscious awareness of the new perspectives.

The ego is a strong force for turning everything into itself, vs. being changed by openly taking in new information. There were times when I was open enough to what I had been holding onto somatically, that the realizations brought through the gift of this work were cognitive and profound. Through some miracle I was ready to have my view of the world change. At other times, as with all shadow work, I felt somewhat uncomfortable, unclear and confused although definitely more alive, as hidden areas of consciousness were given at least some space to move and be felt, even if only partially.

I highly recommend this work to anyone on a path of self knowledge, especially for those whose path has not included an unquestionably somatic component. For those whose self work has included a somatic component, I recommend it just for the pure exploratory fun of it. In either case you'll find it hard work, but I think you'll enjoy the "ride."

THE EMBODIED VOICE

AN INTERVIEW WITH SYLVI ALLI

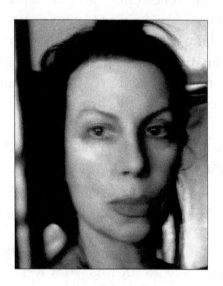

SYLVI ALLI

In 1989, Sylvi began her musical journey into ambient/industrial electronic music and six years later, she began adding her voice experimentation to the mix. This direction led to the development of soundtracks for various dance performance as well as Antero Alli's theatre and cinema projects. She has acted in many of Alli's films and has performed in a number of their paratheatrical productions. Her deep background in Paratheatre (since 1996) has informed her "embodied voice" approach to singing through movement.

The interviewer, Jonnie Gilman is a Seattle-based journalist.

Jonnie Gilman: *What do you mean by "embodied voice"?*

Sylvi Alli: "Embodied voice" is, for me, a voice that is grounded, rooted, in the physical body. In my work, I have come to experience the body as a vessel for the voice to move through and resonate within. There is a noticeable difference in the resonance of a voice initiated from the belly, for example, and a voice initiated from their upper throat. This ties in with where one's awareness lies—are you singing/moving from the belly, or from the head? As a culture, many of us spend the majority of our waking lives "in our head." When the awareness moves further down the body, the vibrational quality of the voice deepens, producing a fuller, richer sound.

I also use the term "authentic voice" in the work that I do. This is the voice that emerges when we let go of the effort of the ego, when we find a place of compassion and acceptance of where we are in the moment, our natural voice, when we shift from being "the singer" to the one "being sung."

JG: *What is your process? How do you help people find their "authentic voice"?*

SA: My work with singers involves a number of levels, some of which are:

BREATH WORK and GROUNDING

I usually begin at the level of breath. Without good breath support, our voices can only strain and flail. Breath work is part of the grounding process that is crucial to this work, as well.

PHYSICAL ENGAGEMENT

The strengthening of physical connection, of "feeling one's body more deeply," is paramount for this work—rendering the body more open for the voice to resonate within. Stretching and core work are employed to increase flexibility and heat; exploration of physical expression encourages new access to the voice.

ENERGIES and SOURCES

Then there is the more mysterious part of the work that involves the person or group actively exploring various energy states and sources, and through this engagement, vocal and physical expression to the source. This level of engagement can run the gamut from subtle shifts, to intense release, to new insights into one's true nature.

TONING and CHANTING

Toning is used in this work for a number of reasons—to connect voice with body, to explore vocal placement, and to express the voice without the added charge of words.

After individual exploration, an opportunity is created to sing as a group. I like teaching chants in this work, mainly for their devotional nature. Once we are opened up to more internal processes, chanting is a wonderful way to bring that energy into a focused expression through the heart center.

JG: In your teaching method you emphasize movement and physicality. What impact does body movement have upon the voice?

SA: Physical movement is utilized in this method primarily to increase one's connection to the body—by increasing flexibility, releasing tension, and raising physical heat. This process creates an environment in which the voice can reach deeper and stronger resonances, and, just as importantly, brings us out of the mental realm, into a purer, more accessible vibrational realm.

JG: Why/how does someone stifle their voice? What are the blocks to being able to sing?

SA: Since I have been doing this work, I have met so many women who share a similar experience of having been discouraged to express themselves vocally. If they were in a choir, for example, they were asked to stand in the back, or just "mouth the words." Women, especially, have traditionally been taught to "keep quiet." These early experiences have had a stifling effect on self-expression, which singing is a form of, further effecting the sense of one's own value or worth.

Even if there was no early trauma of being told to "shut up," there is still the insidious influence of what is culturally accepted as sounding "good." Whether it is that critical voice that says your voice doesn't sound good enough, or the unreachable high standards that come from comparing one's voice to the voice of the latest "pop star de jour," buying into these false beliefs keep us from knowing and developing our true, natural voices.

When we sing from the body, rather than from the mind, another form of "listening" develops—a deeper listening that tunes into the interior landscape. This tends to replace the overly critical type of listening that keeps us separated from the purer essence of vocal expression.

JG: As you work with people who come to you for help with freeing their voice, have you noticed a corresponding transformation of other aspects of their being? Do personalities change?

SA: I have definitely seen this work have repercussions on many levels beyond vocal expression, from an increase in energy and emanation, to being able and willing to assert oneself more, to breaking down old rigidities. When we experience singing from our heart, there is a natural opening there. When we find the courage to sing from our gut, an increase of personal strength can occur.

JG: What are some of the changes you have noticed in the people you have worked with?

SA: One of the most common changes that I see is a lessening of self-consciousness. In one of my Embodied Voice class series there was a woman who, in the beginning, was very resistant to singing alone in front of the other women. At the final class, not only was she excited about singing for the group, she had even written her own song to sing. Also, I have often witnessed rigid ego structures softening in those who have done this work, bringing into being more flexibility and compassion.

JG: Is the desire to sound "pretty" or pleasing a block to vocal expression? Is becoming free from self conscious-ness and concern for outcome a part of the process?

SA: The lessening of self consciousness is a natural out-come of this work. As we strengthen our capacity for self-acceptance and compassion, another faculty of "listening," a deeper listening, takes hold. Greater access to the inner landscape develops through this non-judgmental environ-ment, finding the fertile silence from which all sound arises. There is an aspect to the work that encourages a new way of registering one's voice, where we begin to "feel" our voice rather than "listening to the sound of our voice."

JG: How has your yoga practice and study of North-ern Indian vocal music influenced your teaching?

SA: Having practiced yoga for many years has given me a foundation of physical discipline, as Northern Indian voice training has supported specific vocal development. But neither of these has influenced my embodied voice teaching nearly as much as the work I have done in a group ritual technology called "Paratheatrical Research" led by my partner, Antero Alli. It was through this work that I found a totally new approach to using my voice, and it was this experience that inspired me to further develop this process and share it with others through my group facilitation.

JG: Do you think that singing is an inherent human capability? Can anyone sing?

SA: I believe that if you can speak, you can sing. But in saying this, I have met a few people who seem to be missing the ability to reproduce exact pitch, i.e. "sing in key." So, in the sense of expressing oneself vocally, that is what I mean—beyond what is more as "singing." Perhaps a truer way of putting it is, I feel that anyone who can speak has the ability to express themselves vocally with the singing voice. This does not mean that they will, not everyone is ready or willing to open up to expressing themselves in this way. But essentially, singing is a natural, effortless act.

JG: What has this work taught you? Has it influenced your own expression?

SA: That the more I can "get out of the way," the greater and truer my vocal expression becomes! I used to be a very self-conscious singer. The freedom and joy that I have found through this vocal embodiment process has been immense and has brought with it a greater expression of music "through me."

PEARLS & PERILS OF COURTING THE MUSES

RITUAL JOURNAL ENTRIES, 2010–2019

The idea of "the Muse" and "the Muses" has vexed, haunted and inspired artists, poets, musicians, authors, painters, sculptors and other creatives for aeons. After nine years of Paratheatre work on this theme, I have come to view the Muses phenomena as an autonomous archetype. In these notes, I won't attempt to explain the enigmatic Muse and Muses (sometimes they're plural) but instead share my notes on how it continues to impact my personal, creative, artistic and spiritual life. — Antero Alli

MUSES NEED VESSELS

Though there seem to be certain attributes and conditions the Muses archetype finds more appealing than others, the nature of these qualities can differ for each person or, as I like to look at it, for each *vessel* the Muses choose for their purposes. People don't choose Muses; Muses choose their own vessels. We don't own the Muses. *They are not my Muses or your Muses but* the Muses. The Muses work through us and then discard their vessels when we cease to be useful or appealing to them. Muses run their own impersonal and autonomous agendas beyond the control and comprehension of anyone courting their favor. Note to self: *The Muses can be fussy, fickle entities; don't expect consistency; stay receptive.*

I see three basic types of Muse vessels: *creatives* (those who live creative lives but don't necessarily produce art; almost all children are "creatives"), *artists* (those who produce art and/or call themselves "artists"), and *creative artists* (those whose art develops from living creatively, whether they call themselves "artists" or not). All three types of vessel represent individuals who sometimes project archetypal Muse status onto others by mythologizing anyone who looks or behaves like a Muse to them. Though these psychic projections can initially arouse romantic, erotic, intoxicating and inspiring emotions, they can also lead to disastrous interpersonal relations. What mortal can live up to anyone's exalted Muse ideal? None I have met. Note to self: *One does not marry the Muse. Don't romance or mythologize or worship the Muses.*

The Muse beckons me towards the Unattainable. When the Muse strikes and takes hold, I sometimes feel beside myself, possessed of a kind of madness. Not insanity exactly, more like a joyous, gleeful obsession. Like a moth sputtering around an open flame, my heart flutters, takes flight towards the Impossible, a fever dream inflaming *amour fou.* The inner mounting flames of Muse-inspired passion or obsession can consume everything and everyone in its wake. I lament the broken hearts and ruined lives of all the men, women and children charred by the creative firestorms of my own Muse-projections. I am guilty here. Note to self: *Court the Muses, not as a lover but as an interaction with the Mysteries. Muses are not always kind, wonderful and loving. They can be ruthless, severe and unforgiving.*

Courting the Muses can sometimes feel like falling madly, deeply in love—a delirium ravaging the soul like a rag doll tilt-a-twirling in gale-force winds. And in this feral astral theatre, the Muses witness my little drama with high indifference. No matter how inspiring or stimulating, their influence creates its own unique stresses on the instrument of self. The Muses don't care if I fall sick or suffer pain or collapse and die; they will simply move on to their next available vessel. The Muses don't care what happens to me; they only care about how well their Presence finds expression through their vessels. If I do not care for the health and maintenance of my instrument of self, this vessel, I become useless to the Muses. Note to self: *Treat the Muses with the same high indifference they treat me. Don't care too much. To stay with the Muses, it's my responsibility to maintain the instrument of self; stay healthy.*

APPEALING TO THE MUSES

Confession: I have become a happy love slave to the Muses. Over forty years of creating original works for experimental theatre, music and cinema I have discovered certain conditions I need to maintain in my daily life for the Muses to find me appealing. How to appeal to the Muses? What routines, thought adjustments, and outlooks keep me receptive to the Muses' signals, timings, whispers? For example, I have found that minimizing the word "is" in my thinking, speaking and writing has helped collapse formulaic, over-literalist thinking that shrivels the imagination, the chief conduit for Muse reception. Note to self: *I am not the "creator" but a translator of the Muse's signals. The real payoff for making Art is neither fame or money or love or power; the payoff is realizing my purpose.*

The Muses demand exposure and elimination of "creative buffers"—those habits, beliefs, events and people that impede or diminish critical receptivity. Meeting these demands to stay receptive has made me more socially selective about the company I keep. Some people, no matter how good their intentions may be, distract my process and drain my energy. Muse dialogue is not about talking to myself or confusing the inner critic or conscious mind or ego with the Muse. *Imposter voices!* These Muse interactions are rarely verbal. They're ineffable impressions or silent signals like flames dancing between transpersonal realms beyond my uneventful, low-drama daily life. Note to self: *Soap opera antics and senseless bickering create static that obscures the Muses' signals. Best to keep the human drama onscreen or on the theatrical stage or in the music. Leave the drama out of daily life.*

TESTED BY THE MUSES

The Muses demand respect. I never call them "my Muses"; if they can be owned, they are not Muses but ego trips. I call them *the Muses* for good reason. They come and go on their own accord, on their own schedule and timing. *They are not on my watch; I am on their watch.* When the Muses disappear, I take it as a sign to earn more patience by tending to fallow fields between projects, doing nothing does not have to be a problem. Some fallow field dry spells can last a year or two. Back and forth, between action and inaction, expresses a dynamic balance between the stimulation-oriented sympathetic nervous system and the rest-oriented parasympathetic nervous system. Too much of one or the other can throw the whole system off. Note to self: *My value to the Muses does not depend on constant productivity; periods of rest and recovery are important for restoring receptivity. Only when I am empty can the Muses take notice and make use of me.*

Whenever I become too full of myself—gloating over past successes, achievements, accolades—the Muses are bored to tears and start eyeballing other vessels. I remember times when I was obsessed with some brilliant idea that would unexpectedly appear in somebody else's project. W.T.F.?! Did I wait too long? Why did I not follow through when the idea came to me? Note to self: *Without commitment and follow-through, the best ideas languish in the maze of the mind, lighting and leaving for other vessels. Commitment acts as a force. To stay attractive to the Muses, learn to increase the force and heat of my commitment. Thou shalt not bore the Muses!*

The Muses test my faith whenever I worry about where all the resources will come from to produce my next film or theatre project: the talent, the technology, the passion, the time, the money! The Muses mock all my petty concerns. The Muses know that money is not the same as wealth. The Muses trade in the currency of true wealth of talent, of friendships, of time, of love, of skills, and yes, money—all subcategories of the larger category of True Wealth. Worrying about what I don't have disrespects existence and gratitude for the actual conditions of my life. Respect existence or expect resistance. Gratitude, the chief inlet of True Wealth. Note to self: *Gratitude, not attitude. Without gratitude, I am fucked.*

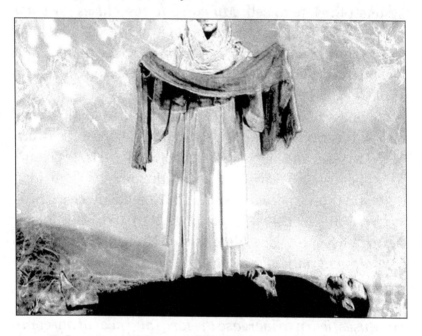

"The Vanishing Field" (2020; Antero Alli)

The Muses dialogue inspired the scripting and production of four feature-length art films: "To Dream of Falling Upwards" (2011), "Flamingos" (2012), "Out of the Woods" (2015) and "The Vanishing Field" (2020), as well as the creation of five paratheatrical productions in Portland (2016–18; photos in back of this book).   — *Antero Alli*

NO-FORM REVELATIONS

IT'S NEVER WHAT I THINK

My ongoing experience and relation with No-Form process have undergone many stages over four decades of Paratheatrical group work. If there's been a consistent thread throughout these stages it's how No-Form has never been what I thought it was. Recently, I discovered how to articulate these stages.   — Antero Alli

FIRST STAGE: RESISTANCE (1977; 5 weeks)

I was initiated into this work after seven years of studying, teaching and performing a style of Mime Theatre combining modern dance and method acting that demanded a high level of control over body, gesture and movement. In this orientation, No-Form was totally inaccessible. I resisted letting go of my highly developed and coveted sense of self-control, a prized technical prowess that also maintained my sense of self, my income, and my status as a performer of physical talent. After five weeks of attempting No-Form, it finally hit me suddenly, like a lightning bolt, and threw me down to the floor, laughing my ass off. A locked door swung open to a bell ringing in an empty sky.

SECOND STATE: RELIGIOUS (1977–1978; 3 months)

Being struck by No-Form acted as a kind of a religious conversion experience. No-Form became for me "the answer to everything," my be-all-end-all truth about Life. I naturally wanted to share the news with the world! For several months, I attempted to convert others to the No-Form experience: *I am Nothing and so are you!* That did not go over well. Like any other religious fanatic, I only ended up alienating myself. Finally, out of sheer futility, I stopped trying to convert others and began my search for another way to cope with my conversion experience.

THIRD STAGE: NOTHING SPECIAL (1979–present day)

During my search, I read *Zen Mind, Beginner's Mind* by Shunryu Suzuki who referred to the No-Form process as *nothing special* (see page 46 in that book). This idea held great appeal for me and helped cool the white hot fire of my religious fervor. No-Form practice in Paratheatrical process became more workman-like. I focused more on the function of No-Form, what it did—*as a trance-induction device and as a tool for trance-dispersion or, for breaking trance*—than No-Form as God. Make trance, break trance. No-Form became more practical, less "religious."

FOURTH STAGE: ESCAPE (1990–1993; 3 years)

During this stage, No-Form became for me a kind of escape, a refuge and sanctuary, from the anxiety and stresses of daily life. Here, No-Form provided a deep sense of safety missing from my life, a meta-place where I could disappear and avoid the static of the out-there world and the toxic default culture at large. However, this escapist tendency proved to be short-lived. It soon became obvious that I could not function in the world the way I wanted to if I was busy hiding in the void. Dwelling in the unmanifest potential state frustrated my needs to manifest certain worldly ambitions, such as creating theatre, writing books or making videos. I was not done with the world and apparently, the world was not done with me yet.

FIFTH STAGE: ACCEPTANCE (1998–present day)

No-Form as "friend." By simple acceptance of No-Form, I developed an ongoing friendship with the fertile Void. A gentle rapport helped me stay receptive, a critical condition for staying creative and close to the Muses, those sources of inspiration guiding my life and my artworks. This deepened capacity for receptivity became a strong value that remains in me to this day, a value that sustains all my creative work, my interpersonal relations, and the realization of my dreams.

SIXTH STAGE: IDENTITY (2008–present day)

No-form as true nature. After three decades of No-Form practice in paratheatrical group work I became increasingly aware of not only a deepening acceptance of and relationship with the fertile Void, but an experience of myself as an expression of the Void—not as any concept or idea but as identity. Void as true nature. When entering No-Form in paratheatrical work, I have only to remember who I am and instantly a deep receptivity opens up. This stage seems to hold an almost infinite capacity for creativity that I cannot see any further stages of the No-Form experience beyond maybe integrating all previous five stages. I'm not counting this as any final arrival; No-Form continues to defy whatever I thought it was or should be.

PerformanceWorks NW (Portland workspace)

POTENTIAL THREATS, DANGERS, SELF-DELUSION

PERILS & PRATFALLS OF LONG-TERM PARATHEATRICAL WORK

What defines "danger" can differ for each person; one person's threat can be another person's excitement. Before starting group work, participants are asked to take a vow to accept full responsibility for their own safety and for exciting their own creative states. If you are unwilling and/or unable to take this vow, it may be best to refrain from doing this work until you are ready to do so. Being accountable for your own safety means that when you register threat of any kind, whether perceived or actual, you agree to do your best to restore your sense of safety in whatever way works for you in a trial by error process. Exciting your own creative states means discovering ways to raise your own energy, to openly express yourself and engage more fluid, spontaneous modes of action, relating and being. This self-accountability vow nurtures personal autonomy and integrity, core values of this work.

PHYSICAL THREAT

Very few physical injuries have occurred over the last forty years I have done this work alone and with many others. Physical dangers are usually caused by careless movement and ignorance of personal boundaries, one's own and others'. Naivete around the limitations of your physical strength, flexibility and stamina can also lead to physical injury in any physically active situation. In this work process, everyone moves at their own pace. Everyone is also responsible for discovering and establishing their own boundaries. This choice-centered "adult" approach to dynamic physical and creative processes significantly minimizes the threat of physical danger.

EMOTIONAL THREAT

This work occurs in an asocial climate where self-work replaces the fulfillment of social needs and wants. When emotional and social needs go unmet, we can feel more insecure around others who are not there to meet our needs. This is why ongoing work in this medium necessitates a support system and social life outside of the workspace. When our emotional and social needs are frustrated, we can feel more needy and, draw more attention to ourselves that can drain group morale and momentum. This work can be highly self-confrontational, exposing rigid beliefs and assumptions that can be upsetting. We can also feel threatened when our inflated self-images and ego structures are deflated when confronting more truth about ourselves. Any confrontation with the archetype of The Self can feel like defeat for the ego. A sense of humor about oneself goes a long way in this work.

PSYCHOLOGICAL THREAT

In this work, the "shadow" aspects of ourselves—what we fear, loathe or avoid about ourselves—can surface to conscious awareness and shock any one-sided ego, or self-image. Our human condition contains a vast spectrum of qualities, colors and attributes. In truth, we are not always "good" or "bad", not always "smart" or "ignorant"; both sides of our nature, light and dark, are equally valid in their own ways. In this work we are exposed to the greater contraries of what Carl Jung called the archetype of The Self; we are both good and bad, smart and ignorant, beautiful and ugly, etc.

> *"The Self embraces not only the conscious but also the unconscious psyche, and is therefore, a personality which we also are. The Self is not only the centre but also the whole circumference which embraces both conscious and unconscious; it is the centre of this totality, just as the ego is the center of consciousness."*
> — Carl Gustav Jung

With increasing Self-exposure, we gain access to the internal landscape of the human condition, expanding the playing fields of creation. However, this consciousness expanding experience requires courage and heart. To live with more truth about ourselves, we must learn to show more acceptance and compassion for our shortcomings and perceived defects; truth without compassion can feel just like cruelty.

As we accept more of our totality, our self-image (i.e., ego) expands and stretches to contain more experience of The Self, more truth. However, just because we can access or embody certain archetypal forces (in a ritual context) does not automatically make us "gods" and "goddesses. Though ego-inflation can be an important stage in the development of personality, becoming too full of ourselves can also diminish the receptivity necessary for staying creative. Excessive ego-inflation can also alienate us with self-important, obnoxious behavior and toxic attitudes. Once deflated any big ego can drop down to "body size" through a deepening commitment to no-form practice. *It's tough being a bighead when deep down we know we are nothing.*

SPIRITUAL THREAT

Ongoing work in this paratheatre medium stimulates the sympathetic function of the Central Nervous System (CNS). This process activates the energetic body, the subtle chakra system and its corresponding endocrine glands. When over-stimulated, we may suffer insomnia after a night's ritual session ends. Excess electromagnetism can be discharged by deepening your no-form practice after each and every ritual. Another safe way to neutralize excess electromagnetic charge is soaking 10–20 minutes in an Epsom Salt bath (using one cup Epsom salts per 100 pounds of body weight and showering afterward).

Spiritual crisis can occur with any spontaneous epiphany exposing a loss of connection or faith in God or Source and/or a collapsing belief system. This shock can trigger an *epistemological crisis,* causing us to question our core values and beliefs, shaking the very foundation of our being. When our belief systems are exposed as obsolete, we naturally feel anxious. Everyone has their own "uncertainty threshold," of how much uncertainty we can tolerate before anxiety sets in. When we find ways to manage the force of our own anxiety, we can permit more uncertainty. One way to manage anxiety is to reframe uncertainty as a creative state. Permitting more uncertainty opens us to new experiences and new ways of responding to our experiences.

THE POTENTIAL FOR SELF-DELUSION

It's been my experience so far that the potential for self-delusion comes with any self-work that triggers the expression of autonomous forces from the Unconscious into the conscious ego. Paratheatre offers a rich palate of pathways and techniques for accessing the internal land-scape in sometimes cathartic ways. With practice, these processes can arouse deep feelings, insights, revelations and epiphanies about oneself and one's place in the cos-mos. However, any experience—*no matter how profound at the time*—can easily vanish as fading memories if they are not applied and integrated into daily life.

Any deeply-charged subjective experiences can lead to self-delusion if we assume the experience was enough to significantly change our lives; sometimes it can, some-times it can't. Without consistent follow-through and application of our realizations, we can easily become entranced by the spell of thinking we are doing something important when, in fact, we are only thinking ABOUT doing something important. *What actually gets done is self-delusion.* Without integrating our insights into the larger fabric of our life beyond the workspace, we set up a delusory escapist relationship with paratheatre itself. When we approach ritual work with the intention or hope of escaping the drudgery of mundane existence, we risk a kind of presbyterian milktoast approach to transformative work.

THE "POOR BABY" SYNDROME

Sometimes paratheatre work can ignite *an epistemological crisis* where our current values are exposed as meaningless, trivial, obsolete or worthless. This crisis can sometimes lead to an emotional downward spiral of despair. When we cannot stop condemning ourselves for failing to live up to the bloated expectations of our ego ideals, we can suffer the self-importance of negative ego-inflation. We may blame our failure on society or on Republicans! No matter what the cause or the symptoms, when our spirit is crushed by self-imposed negative attitudes and beliefs, we play the victim. *Poor baby!*

Since paratheatre work demands a healthy ego and a supple energetic body, it may be difficult to do this work in a state of negative inflation or low emotional energy. It can be like trying to drive a car with an empty tank. Without an ample supply of emotional energy, paratheatre turns rote, contrived or superficially "play-acted." To break the trance of the Victim archetype, the Poor Baby syndrome must be exposed, defused and dismantled. This can occur in any ritual that gives expression to the Victim archetype, so it can then be played out, embraced and released.

It may be natural to feel inadequate in the face of any hurdle we perceive as insurmountable. However, feelings of helplessness and inadequacy are not the same as being helpless. When negative emotions are mistakenly identified with as absolutes, we become self-deluded. Emotions are not absolute; *they just feel absolute.* When over-emphasized, negative emotions diminish the being; our authentic self shrinks. A negative being simply means *an absence of being*—a non-entity.

THE MESSY MESSIANIC COMPLEX

Conscious surrender to, and embodiment of, archetypal energies—*an important ritual talent*—can naturally result in positive inflation of ego, or a big self-image. We can feel like "gods and goddesses" and believe that we are. Positive ego inflation can express a natural phase of ego development. As we open up to more aspects of The Self, we discover the inherent contraries of our true nature—we are good enough to be bad, intelligent enough to confess ignorance, independent enough to embrace dependencies, strong enough to feel weak. Embracing internal contraries nurtures an alchemical transformation within *the Vas Hermeticum of the Body itself.*

Positive ego inflation becomes excessive when we confuse the ego for The Self and forget that ego expresses one aspect of The Self; ego is subordinate to the archetype of Self. When we confuse ego for The Self, self-delusion enflames a messy messianic complex of obnoxious self-importance and entitlement—*attitudes, behaviors, beliefs and ideas of excessive narcissism.* We become more easily offended and/or lose a sense of humor about ourselves. We erroneously expect others to take us as seriously as we take ourselves. Sometimes these internal expectations find support in our squads of Yes Men and Yes Women who buy into our fantasy and enable our self-delusion. You want out of this mess? Play the fool. Get over yourself. Blow your cover. Be vulnerable. Re-discover the seriousness of a child at play. Go to clown school.

RELIGIOUS CONVERSION EXPERIENCE

Another symptom of the messianic complex manifests as a compulsion to convert others to beliefs we falsely assume as absolutes. As this self-delusion escalates, the ego bloats by identifying itself as a kind of master or savior figure stridently rallying others behind its bloated cause. These conversion tactics often express a naive reflex following any genuine religious conversion experience. When we experience God in whatever form or shape, we naturally want to share the God experience with others, whatever that God is. We humans have a talent for making a religion out of almost anything and rallying others around our altars and churches.

Effective strategies to defuse the positive inflation of the Messianic complex can be found in any ego-corrosive actions where we place ourselves in service to others. This can take any number of forms, from actions that alleviate the suffering of others to assisting those who cannot help themselves to performing hard physical labor for the benefit of another. Ego-corrosive actions, however, are not for everybody. Those with more fragile egos or who cannot endure or stomach the suffering of others may not find it as useful.

ON BREAKING CERTITUDE TRANCE

Self-delusion can also result from suffering the illusion of excessive certainty. We delude ourselves after fixating on any picture, image, idea, vision, belief, or assumption as an absolute in our minds. The self-deluded mind confuses opinions for facts and fantasy for reality. Mental fixation can be defused by learning to relax the search for meaning and by allowing things to happen without trying to control the outcome.

To break the trance of excessive certitude, permit more uncertainty. Live a day without a self-image, or a day without fixating on any idea of who you are or should be. Breathe in the rare air of a concept-free zone.

closure

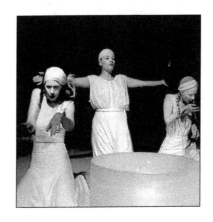

5

UNDOING THE WORLD

MANIFESTO, PARTS 1–5

Part 1: Culture, Verticality, The Asocial

The following five-part manifesto was written, updated and rewritten over fifteen years of group paratheatrical research. It's included here to clarify the underlying principles, methods and discoveries that occurred over this period, as well as, to share my reflections on the larger contexts of sociopolitical trends. This manifesto does not posit any absolute answers or final arrivals but rather the fruition of a work in progress.   — Antero Alli

ON CULTURE

One of my mentors, Christopher S. Hyatt, suggested that culture may be nothing more or less than the ongoing results of daily interactions between human DNA and geography. I came to understand his big picture vision as what happens when a given tribe dwells within any given bioregion where a distinct culture develops through its ongoing interaction with the native food resources, power fields, the land and weather patterns sustaining them there. Mountain ranges, deserts, shorelines, valleys and forests all carry distinct powers of influence shaping the daily lives and souls of the people living there—what they eat, the artifacts they create, and the technology (tools) they need to survive within this complex Planet/People weave we call "culture."

When we take pride in "our" culture or believe we can "create" culture, a delusional field is ignited obscuring the true source of culture. Nobody owns culture; we are more likely owned by the culture we live in. Culture as the ongoing interplay between human genes and geography develops organically. Nobody creates culture. We are more likely 'created' by culture. At best we can contribute to and maybe even advance a culture; at worst, we can corrupt and destroy it. Any culture corrupts when it becomes excessively anthropocentric and loses touch with its vitalizing sources in the geocentric pulse of the living earth.

We live in an era of dying cultures. To survive, any culture or subculture must turn to those rituals and traditions that sustain it. Any human culture achieves longevity by the success of its sustaining rituals, how well we are feeding the planet, and how well we are being fed by the planet. Sustaining rituals return us to the primordial interaction with our immediate womb environment through soulful communion and communication with the planetary entity. These sustaining rituals cannot be understood or proven by any empirical, literalist mindset. However, our primordial contact with planetary forces can be experienced firsthand through intuitive resonance with the Earth as a living entity *that has incarnated as our planet. The planet is not dying; the egocentric cultures feeding off of the planet are dying.*

Some geomantic power fields and planetary hotspots express innately charged conflict zones where highly volatile energies dwell and erupt without warning: earth-quakes, tsunamis, volcanos, hurricanes, tornados, lightning strikes, landslides. The underlying causes of human conflict, violence and warfare may run deeper than bloodlust for revenge, money, power, oil and religion. In these conflict zones, we may be unconsciously acting as conduits, vessels, for the eruptions of feral geomantic forces innate to the region we live in. There are also geomantic leylines and electromagnetic fields expressing a deep harmony that supports the development of more harmonious cultures and the people that inhabit these regions.

We act on culture and are acted on by culture. Over time—decades, centuries, aeons—this genes/geography interplay crystallizes into symbols, languages and artifacts that encode, encrypt and transmit the characteristics of each distinct cultural identity. Cultures developing in the Himalayan mountains will differ from cultures stimulated along the shorelines of southern India or the Sonoran deserts of Mexico or the lush Amazon river basin or the Cascadian forests of the Pacific Northwest. Each unique bioregion informs the nature of its tribe's religions, arts, mythologies, commerce, education, language, community rituals, and values. Though each culture maintains its own distinct signature and appearance by its unique sustaining rituals and traditions, all cultures are linked by the universal molecular language of DNA; we are all human beings living and dying on the same planet.

ON THEATRE AND THE PARATHEATRICAL

Theatre acts as one of many sustaining rituals keeping a culture alive. As with any sustaining ritual, theatre must evolve and change over time to meet the growing needs and values of the era, the people, and their environment. Like a snake shedding old skin, any culture molts and grows by outgrowing itself. Any theatre that cannot outgrow itself ceases to function as a vital sustaining ritual. For theatre to remain vital, a kind of Paratheatre must be developed and implemented to dismantle stagnant work habits frustrating creative response. Paratheatre—*in the theatre but not of it*—provides a context set apart from theatre to experiment with excavating the internal landscape of autonomous forces in the Body for vital and spontaneous movements, gestures, vocalizations, actions and interactions—in a kind of *archeology of the soul.*

This excavation process starts with releasing the pressure to perform and replacing it with self-created pressures to increase personal commitment to sources of energy, impulses, power and grace within the Body itself. This redirection of commitment, from external to internal, opens the door to our innate verticality—*what can be experienced as energy/information flowing down from above and up from below, as a vertical column running up and down the spine.* Alignment with our innate verticality initiates receptivity towards engaging and expressing *the Body as the living embodiment of the so-called Subconscious mind.*

"With verticality the point is not to renounce part of our nature; all should retain its natural place: the body, the heart, the head, something that is 'under our feet' and something that is 'over the head.' All like a vertical line, and this verticality should be held taut between organicity and the awareness. Awareness means the consciousness which is not linked to language (the machine for thinking), but to Presence."

— Jerzy Grotowski

VERTICALITY, ASOCIAL INTENT, THE ARCHETYPE OF SELF

Groups create bonds of shared acceptance, support and belonging through community-building social events. However these social bonds can also inhibit or frustrate the expression of true feelings and spontaneous responses which frustrates creativity. When a given group becomes preoccupied with maintaining their social personas and meeting their social needs—*for friendship, courtship, belonging, approval, security, status, etc.*—this group begins feeding horizontally-oriented social needs and the sense of verticality is quickly lost or was never established in the first place.

The experience of verticality can be accessed in an asocial work climate. Implementing an asocial intent starts with realizing our non-responsibility to others in the workspace. This shift from external to internal dependence replaces social considerations with an active discovery of our most honest, spontaneous and authentic responses. Without this adjustment, the "default" conditioning of our local culture's socialization 'programs' can easily dominate the tone of any group interaction and corrupts the quality of paratheatrical work with social clichés and conditioned reactions. Actualizing an asocial intent naturally frustrates social compulsions and needs to bind social agreements. Social needs are obviously important but are best met outside of the workspace. By relaxing our social agendas and motivations, we can begin sourcing the internal landscape of autonomous forces in a somatic, visceral expression of what Carl Jung calls Active Imagination *for making the Unconscious, conscious*. This starts the process of Self-initiation through interacting with the centralizing archetype of The Self.

> *"The Self is a quantity that is supra ordinate to the conscious ego. It embraces not only the conscious but also the unconscious psyche, and is therefore, so to speak, a personality which we also are. The Self is not only the centre but also the whole circumference which embraces both conscious and unconscious; it is the centre of this totality, just as the ego is the center of consciousness."*
> — Carl Jung, *Two Essays on Analytical Psychology*

Part 2: Integrity Loss & Recovery
commitment, sacrifice, the impersonal culture

SELF-TRUST AND THE FORCE OF COMMITMENT

No such thing as self-improvement. You cannot improve who you are; you already are who you are. You are not some kind of apprentice to yourself who will someday, with enough "self-improvement," become the real you. It is too late for that. You can wake up to who you are and accept yourself or, keep trying to improve this thing called "self," whatever that is. Who are you beyond your beliefs, assumptions, self-images and ideas of who you are? Certain habits and behaviors can certainly be corrected and "improved" but we'd be mistaken to assume identity there. You are not only more than you think, you are more than you *can* think.

The aim of paratheatrical work is to discover our firsthand experience as a source of authority, integrity and autonomy. This inner work starts with increasing the force of our self-commitment. This means becoming fully accountable for our experiences, choices, actions and their consequences. Before self-commitment can be increased, it may be necessary to expose any doubts, distrust, or negation of firsthand experience as an authority source. Perhaps we were raised by a family or schools that dismissed personal experience as too subjective to be relied on as a barometer of truth. If so, this dismissal of your own experience may have damaged the self-trust essential to even having an experience. Trusting firsthand experience as an authority source demands a time-intensive process of testing its legitimacy for ourselves. Once enough self-trust can be earned and established, we are more free to interact with others and the world from a greater sense of personal integrity. With enough self-trust, more reality-based relationships can develop free of wanting approval or acceptance for what we already know from firsthand experience.

SACRIFICE; THE LIFE & DEATH WISHES

Any act of true sacrifice unleashes torrents of creative and psychic force. Something can only be a true sacrifice if what we are asked to give up has become near and dear to our hearts. Releasing our attachment to cherished objects, possessions, relationships, jobs, dreams and goals unleashes the torrent of forces invested in them. True sacrifice tills the ground of our being for seeds of new behavior, new ideas, new beliefs, new habits and new rituals.

This force of self-commitment is rooted in our survival instincts for how committed we are to being on the planet. If you are still alive and breathing, some part of you remains committed to being on the planet. Our daily lives are shaped by deeper unconscious forces that I call *the death-wish and the life-wish.* If you feel grave doubt or are deeply conflicted about being on the planet, the death-wish is winning. When you are more fully committed to being on the planet, the life-wish dominates. These contrary forces of regeneration and degeneration express the underlying existing conditions of our lives. Whatever we choose to align ourselves with determines the quality and nature of our fates. A metaphor comes to mind—*if fate is in the cards, destiny is how they're played.*

What makes our lives worth living, without which our lives would not be worth living? At some point in our lives, we face what we are living for: *life or death.* Until then, we are second-guessing our reasons for being. The death-wish and life-wish express contrary dynamics within the totality of our human nature; they are not separated at root. Each possesses a function in relation to the whole. Sometimes, we benefit when certain habits or behaviors are allowed to die off; the death-wish becomes relevant! Other times, certain productive areas in our lives suffer weakness or insecurity; committing to the life-wish can resuscitate them.

THE IMPERSONAL NATURE OF CULTURE

Integrity loss is not always a personal problem; it is not entirely our fault if we lack the power of follow-through. We live in an era where integrity loss expresses an impersonal cultural casualty common to any hyper-materialistic, death-ignorant consumerist society fractured by spiritual bankruptcy. Many of us endure this spiritual damage as a private burden we carry for the impersonal culture of society. Even though this damage may not actually be personal to us—*who can take credit?*—many of us mistakenly shoulder the burden of impersonal culture as a personal cause. *What a complete waste of time and energy!* The impersonal culture of society does not, cannot, care about the person. Society at large acts like a corporation that uses the person to advance its impersonal machinations and agendas. *The impersonal culture at large is not your friend.*

Those who drop the impersonal burden of this cultural guilt do not become free of suffering. They become free of the impersonal social culture of suffering that depersonalizes the populace. Only after we embrace the honest burden of our own existence can we know the futility of trying to save the tragedy of the world. When we are fully accountable for our own suffering, we are less likely to believe we are accountable for saving the world. The world does not need saving. The world is full of people who need saving from themselves. Exceptions include those raising children who cannot be accountable for their own survival and those caring for the elderly, the sick, and the dying.

Rejecting the impersonal culture of guilt does not mean shying away from helping others. It means becoming more aware of how we actually can and cannot help another. Not everyone needs or wants to be saved or awakened from their cocooning trance of impersonal cultural identification. Try breaking the spell of anyone resigned to the comfort of spiritual sleep and you may face the gnashing of teeth, the bearing of claws. Sometimes, naive gestures of helping others can be experienced as offensive, invasive, or annoying to those being "helped." If we are to actually assist others, we must first relax our personal agendas to discover more truth about their values, history, allegiances and beliefs. Otherwise, we may be simply imposing our so-called help and alienate ourselves and others in the process.

Not all suffering is meaningful. Suffering becomes meaningless when it results in a more meaningless life. Meaningful suffering results in a more meaningful life. How to tell the difference? Look to the results of your suffering to determine whether it's actually relevant or pointless. Self-created suffering—*over-thinking, courtship compulsion, self-pity, nonstop complaining*—can render our lives meaningless. Suffering that builds character, compassion and strength renders our lives with more meaning. Meaningful suffering demands an honest confrontation with the existing conditions of our actual (not ideal) lives, i.e., not the life we wanted or believed we should or could have had, if only things were different. No—I'm talking about your actual life.

Respect existence or expect resistance. A living mystery pulses within the heart of existence—that we exist at all is a mystery! By exposing and surrendering ourselves to the existing conditions of our lives, a dimension of mystery can be penetrated and experienced firsthand. At some point, we may even become aware that we are this mystery and we embody it. *Become the mystery.*

Part 3: The Performer/Audience Romance
need for love, talent & skill, the total act, No-Form

FALLING IN LOVE WITH WHAT

The torrid romance of audience/performer dynamics is fraught with mystery, anticipation and insecurity. The tremulous rush of stage fright does not come from any promise of long-term relationship but the spine-tingling prospect of an eternal one-night stand. Theatrical conventions of distance (the fourth wall), talent and skill naturally separate performers and audience, a separation sealed by post-performance audience applause. The audience/performer power dynamic tips and sways with fickle electricity; one night we're up and on, the next night we're down and out. As with any one-night stand, the audience/performer romance remains unpredictable and most performers would not have it any other way.

Can real connection between performer and an audience actually occur? Yes and no. Real connection between audience and performer may not be possible through any direct attack—presentational confrontations where the performer directly manipulates and/or emotionally assaults the audience. Whether it's via seduction, performer charisma, or the performers' "need to please, be liked, or to impress others"—or the more aggressive "in your face" assaults of Artaud's Theatre of Cruelty or Julian Beck's Living Theatre—direct attack theatre often fails to achieve any real connection beyond sledgehammer dents and crashes. Though this direct attack approach can sometimes prove effective as political theatre, historically it has consistently failed to achieve its social utopian ideals of "awakening the sleeping masses" or "saving or changing the world."

A PERFORMER'S NEED FOR LOVE

No matter how great a given performance, the audience can only love the performance but not the person performing it, unless they are performing as themselves and not a character. Everyone needs and deserves love but that's not what the audience can offer. Confusing audience applause for love is like feasting on popcorn; you bloat and stay hungry for more popcorn. As a cultural entity, the audience has been conditioned by centuries of tradition to act as a passive, receptive vessel for the stimulation of their own impressions, emotions, ideas, beliefs and reactions to performances presented onstage or onscreen. The audience applauds a performance for arousing their own passions, thoughts, views and sense of identification—in short, for arousing their own humanity. When any performance achieves this arousal, the audience responds with applause, praise, admiration and respect. But not love. Oh, we hear them say, "I absolutely love your show"... "What an amazing performance"... "LOVE your work" and so on, but all these affects quickly fade. Audiences can be fickle; one night they're warm and responsive and the next night they're aloof and we never hear from them again.

Those who fall for "audience love" are fated to wander and chase the hungry ghost high of leap-frogging from production to production, from film to film, without taking any significant breaks to breathe, to live, to actually love and be loved. Attempting to meet your need for personal love in any audience-defined medium may be the worst reason to become an actor or a performer. Better to find someone to love (and to love you) and then, decide why you want to perform. If you can't find someone to love, love yourself like there's no tomorrow. Or if you are so graced, turn to God for the unconditional love no human can be expected to provide and then, share this spiritual presence with the world. Become the love that you seek. Love is never what we think. Love is the law, the crime that creates and breaks the law.

THE TOTAL ACT—CAPACITY FOR RESONANCE

Why do we perform? If we are to make real connection with the audience, the will to perform must be liberated from all externally-driven considerations such as seeking acceptance, pleasing others, trying to impress the director, getting attention, love or approval, or seeking external acceptance for our talents, skills and abilities. Only when the will to perform is emancipated from external social approval mechanisms can we become aligned with what Jerzy Grotowski calls *"the total act."*

Performance of the total act requires development of an internal faculty of resonance, an intuitive capacity for knowing truth. Resonance requires no understanding, forethought, or plan. We either resonate with a given direction or state or we do not. When we lose this resonating capacity, we suffer indecision and can be plagued by vagueness of direction or over-thinking. Whenever we can fully commit to the visceral and spiritual resonances within us, a ripple effect occurs. Like a stone dropped in a calm pool of water, our personal resonances indirectly stir similar resonances in others and in the audience. This mutual interaction of resonances relies on the performer's total commitment to their own visceral and spiritual sources which, in turn, trigger audience resonances. In this way, the audience experiences an amplification of their own presence and not just the impact of a performer's force, or will, or charisma. After such a performance, the audience leaves exalted and amplified, as if they are leaving with more of themselves than when they arrived.

How can we cultivate a deeper capacity for resonance? A violin produces resonant tones due to its empty chamber; a violin stuffed with cotton becomes muted. To increase our internal resonating capacity, we must learn how to cultivate a kind of "empty chamber" within the instrument of the self. If we are stuffed with ideas, beliefs, techniques and knowledge, our capacity for internal resonance quickly diminishes. The creation of internal space requires a process of "undoing" or emptying. There are many ways to initiate this process of undoing. The most direct and simple approach I have discovered and used in paratheatre is a method borrowed from Zen meditation that I call No-Form. In paratheatre, it's practiced in a standing posture, rather than traditional Zazen sitting meditation; one cannot move very far while sitting. The aim of this No-Form stance is to cultivate enough internal receptivity to detect and then, be acted on by autonomous forces in the body/psyche. By engaging and expressing these forces, we allow their presence to act through us as vessels in spontaneous movement, sound, gesture and actions.

THE UNDOING METHOD OF NO-FORM

Though No-Form represents a very direct and simple process, it can also be difficult and frustrating for anyone burdened by over-thinking, compulsive rationalization, and excessive self-analysis. The Inner Critic and the Ego Ideal naturally resist the prospect of being nothing. Other impediments to No-Form include: identification with self-images, preconceptions, ideals, beliefs, over-confidence and excessive certitudes. No-Form can be experienced as a kind of intimacy with Void, a comfort around being nothing...of being nobody.

No-Form can be approached in any standing posture of balance resulting in a position of vertical rest—standing with minimal effort—and supporting a state of emptying or internal receptivity. The breath is focused on the exhale, allowing the inhale to occur by reflex. Mentally, we relax the desire to control and the desire to control the outcome or any appearance of our expression.

No-Form acts to charge a ritual to engage the body's vital forces and then to discharge these forces after each ritual or performance. In this way, No-Form serves a double function as a receptivity point to creative energy and then, as a discharging point to release whatever energies were engaged. It's like an on/off switch to our creative engines. Some performers seem to be "on" all the time, as if they never found the "off" switch. No-Form practice allows us to turn the creative engines on and off according to our needs. In this way, we are free to use our talents and skills as tools, instead of being owned by them. We no longer need to fear losing access to our creative sources or diminishing our talents when we know how to turn our creative engines on and off.

THE W.N.S. (WAYNE NEWTON SYNDROME)

The audience/performer dynamic expresses an inherent imbalance. As performers, we're onstage because we exhibit, or should exhibit, more talent and skill than the audience that has paid to see us. The audience expects to be entertained and enlightened to some aspect of their lives and of their humanity. The audience arrives looking to be informed, stimulated and amused. Performers are paid to control the communication in whatever medium they're working in; performers call the shots, must call the shots. When the actors take charge and do their job, theatre happens. There is a difference, however, between theatre that just gets the job done and *theatre that changes lives.*

Performers of theatre that changes lives must continually develop their craft in very specific and precise ways. Though these ways may differ for each performer, it starts with making choices on projects that stretch and expand our existing skill sets and talents. Without consistently challenging ourselves, performers can slip into plateaus of redundancy and stagnation by getting paid for repeating what they already know and what they do best. Without consistent challenges, artists can easily sink into a quagmire of inertia; existing talents wither, corrupt, fritter away. We become more tourist than artist, more mimic than creator, more spectacle than substance.

The Universal Patron Saint of Show Biz Glitz, Wayne "Mr. Las Vegas" Newton, demonstrates the fate awaiting those who only perform what they do best. Don't get me wrong. Mr. Newton is a wonderful and talented performer. He just does what he does over and over and over and over, again...and gets paid handsomely for it...

> *"I'm still doing the kind of shows I've always done and I can tell you one thing: people may leave one of my shows disliking Wayne Newton, but they've never walked out saying, 'He didn't work hard for us' or 'He didn't give us our money's worth.'"*
> — Wayne Newton

TALENT AND SKILL

Talent demonstrates a fluid capacity for gaining access and expression of the internal landscape in a spirit of constant discovery. Skill refers to a dexterity for articulating the internal landscape through externally recognizable forms, symbols, images, speech and structures. Skill shows precision and clarity of form; talent shows spontaneity and "spirit" in action. Through talent we experience the presence and energy of creative force of an artist. With skill, we experience virtuosity, technique and a clear sense of design and form. Artists and performers often demonstrate an imbalance between talent and skill. Too much spontaneity can overwhelm skill, just as too much structure can crimp talent.

Striking a dynamic balance between talent and skill is the aim of any committed artist and/or performer. The more exceptional the performer, the higher the integration of talent and skill. Though talent cannot really be taught, it can be nurtured by encouraging total freedom of self-expression. Skill, however, can be learned by consistent application of method and the refinement of technical dexterity. As talent and skill cohere at higher and higher levels, High Art occurs. Talent in paratheatre refers to an elastic capacity for accessing sources in the body itself, of mining the body for veins of autonomous forces, images, emotion, sensation and the deeper complexes and numinous archetypes of the personal and collective Unconscious—*the inner actions of source-work or sourcing.* Skill in paratheatre refers to the precision of expression and articulation of source-work. Paratheatre skills can be developed by an ongoing practice of paratheatre techniques (see "Trigger Methods").

Part 4: Self-Observation and Ego
identity, contraries, the emotional plague

THE MYSTERY OF IDENTITY

Who are you, really? Are you your name? Are you the offspring of your parents and the genetic link to the future of your ancestral gene pool? Are you the collection of your habits, fears, desires, beliefs, ideas and needs? Are you a figment of your imagination, a dreamer dreaming yourself into existence? Are you what you were hoping for? Beyond all these scenarios, parental and genetic influences, education and philosophical ideas and beliefs, *who are you really?*

"Ego", as the term is used here, refers to any emotional investment and attachment to a self-image. Ego as self-image; big ego as big self-image. Can you distinguish an "image" of who you are from the experience of who you are—before any labels were imposed on that experience? A strong ego is not the same as a big ego that feeds on any inflated, one-sided idea or image of ourselves; big egos express brittle states of psychological rigidity. Strong egos are flexible and at ease in the heart of contradiction, openly embodying the contraries of our universal human condition.

Ego is subordinate to, and created by, The Self, what Jung calls the centralizing archetype of The Self. When the part (ego) is confused for the whole (The Self), the ego becomes "bedeviled." Ego is not the devil but identifying with ego can be vexing. Who has not experienced creative shutdown—*our so-called "creative blocks"*—after falsely assuming credit for what we never truly created or was never truly ours to claim? *We are all imposters!* Why not openly expose the Imposter within us and its social mask, the Poseur? No shame in confession; no crime in being unknown to oneself. Replace the antiquated adage of "Know Thyself" with...*Now Thyself.*

Allowing and embracing contraries within our human nature is an exercise in psychological freedom—freedom from the oppression of a one-sided self-image. For example, if we are enamored by the self-image of being strong, look to your weaknesses to balance your ego. If you are in love with the self-image of independence, are you independent enough to be dependent? If you covet an ego of intelligence, are you smart enough to confess ignorance? If you pride yourself as a "radical person," are you radical enough to be conservative? Embracing our contraries supports a more flexible ego structure.

When the ego is aligned with The Self, we start to experience ourselves as an expression of a larger, changing whole, and can act as vessels for the expression of The Self. As the archetype of Self is accessed, sourced and expressed, we encounter contraries innate to our human nature: we are weak and strong, stupid and intelligent, beautiful and ugly, good and evil. However, it may not be enough to continually expose more truth about ourselves and each other. Truth without self-compassion can feel like cruelty. As empathy for ourselves and for others develops, the narcissism trap can be minimized and sometimes, bypassed. A little narcissism goes a long way and empathy keeps that in check.

THE EMOTIONAL PLAGUE

During the 2020 Plague of Covid, another invisible plague spreads across the land. "The emotional plague," a term coined by Dr. Wilhelm Reich, refers to the "irrational insistence on beliefs and ideas that depend on dissociation of mind from body." This body/mind fissure has been historically dramatized in any religion that maintains this dissociative belief. In the modern era, the emotional plague is sustained by mass projection of vital physical, emotional, psychic and sexual energy into the absorbent mediums of the internet, VR technology, video games, mass media advertising and television. The emotional plague is sustained whenever the virtual is mistaken for the actual, when confusing talk for action, when ideas and ideals are confused for the realities they symbolize, when we are eating the menu instead of the meal.

Two modern-day symptoms of the emotional plague in the current Hypermedia Era: 1) an increasing trend towards de-personalization, homogenization and gentrification and 2) a steadily decreasing capacity for direct experience.

As we lose trust and faith in the legitimacy of firsthand experience, we can naturally become more vulnerable and compliant to the dictates of external sources of authority and its moral codes of obedience and punishment. Without enough trust in our own innate sensibilities, intuitions and instincts we lose touch with our own internal compass. We lose the capacity to distinguish the real from the illusory, the true from the false, and what's right from what's wrong. Without self-trust, we remain as timid children dependent on parental approval and guidance for how we live, work, procreate, domesticate and die.

What is real and what is an illusion? Do you know? Do you care? If you don't know and can say so, you are probably waking up. If you don't know and/or don't care, don't bother; you are probably asleep. It doesn't care either and you will soon be assimilated, if you have not already been consumed by the toxic emotional plague. If you have come to know what's real in life, dare to live by the dictates of your truth. Your example acts as a beacon for those lost at sea struggling to keep their heads above water on the slow-mo shipwreck of the dying cultures at large.

Part 5: Initiation Never Ends
a bridge between worlds;
restoring the dreaming power

ON THE BRIDGE BETWEEN WORLDS

The most challenging aspect of paratheatrical work may be the integration of its results into daily life experiences. Insights, realizations and epiphanies erupting in paratheatrical processes can disappear if they cannot find life beyond the workspace. Without the application of "Lab" insights into the daily, their rarified moments quickly dissipate like fading photographs. For this work to have any lasting influence and value, we must find ways to build and maintain a kind of bridge between worlds— *between the internal landscape of the soul and the external world of daily life*—between the infinite and finite dimensions of existence. How to arouse ecstatic moments amidst day to day toil and drudgery? Can we find No-Form when we're snagged into someone else's soap opera melodramatics? Can we engage verticality in the face of political insanity and corruption? Questions worth addressing.

We humans have always sought out and invented new ways to alleviate boredom and get high and attempt escape from the banality and tedium of existence. Many escape attempts often lead to dispersion and self-destruction, where no true escape happens at all. If this escapist compulsion is innate to the human condition, how can we actually escape? Escapism itself does not seem to be the real problem. The real problem looks more like a naive assumption that we can escape from reality. Nobody escapes from reality. To truly escape, we must find ways to shift the context of escape, from trying to escape from reality towards escaping into reality, into the very heart of the human condition. Escaping into the existing conditions of our lives, rather than away from them, we stand a better chance to tap the pulse of mystery beating at the very heart of existence itself.

At first, this escape into reality may seem impossible and even undesirable. Why would anyone want to pass into and through the wretchedness of mundane existence? This seemingly impossible task demands a certain kind of power, a power that does not originate in any Nietzschean personal "will to power" but a deeper power within our psyches, in our Body, that's drained by unconscious habits of power loss. Maintaining the bridge between worlds requires an exposure and knowledge of habits that drain *the power of dreaming*, a power emanating from the cosmos that we are expressions of.

When we wake up to how we are losing power, we are faced with the choice to minimize or eliminate the drainage points in our lives or keep suffering from power loss. Self-imposed habits of power loss can be self-corrected. Some sources of power loss are imposed on us by others and some come from the dominator culture at large and these require different strategies. Once our power drains are exposed and released, the power of dreaming returns on its own volition. Nothing else has to be done. Remove the drains and the dreaming power returns of itself. This power is not personal, it's not of our personal will; it expresses the cosmos itself. Restoring this dreaming power empowers the bridge between worlds. Maintaining this bridge between worlds must continue as an ongoing ritual of Self-initiation. Like any bridge, new cracks can appear and must be mended. Unattended, new power drains can weaken this bridge. We can fall back and get lost in our own worlds or fall out of ourselves and get eaten by the world.

How the Dreaming Power is Drained

Perhaps the two greatest drains to the dreaming power are: 1) The Poor Baby and 2) Courtship Compulsion. Both drainage points diminish and ravage the energetic body, the chief conduit for the power of dreaming. *The Poor Baby Syndrome corrodes the will.* This power drain is maintained by self-pity and the immature refusal to accept one's flaws, shortcomings and inadequacies. It can manifest as self-denial, constant complaining and whining about feeling "not enough." *Poor Baby!* When afflicted by the Poor Baby Syndrome, we can become as emotional vampyres feeding off the sympathy of others while hosting pity parties in private or commiserating with other Poor Babies. This self-victimizing habit shrinks the decision-making muscle, resulting in the self-created anguish of indecision. The mass culture of advertising feeds and controls the Poor Baby Syndrome by appealing to the unmet needs of the emotionally immature consumer, i.e., *you are not enough without our product!*

Self-denial sustains the Poor Baby. Defusing the Victim archetype starts by learning to accept yourself, warts and all. As self-accountability increases, acceptance eventually replaces self-denial as a powerful foundation of self-support. However, this may be easier said than done. Facing the internal ravages of this power loss can be painful and embarrassing and may require professional therapy if the damage has become too overwhelming for Poor Baby's fragile ego structure.

Taking everything personally fattens the Victim. If you are easily offended, perhaps you suffer from excessive self-importance or delusions of entitlement. This can occur through positive or negative ego-inflation. Unless you're creating a Clown character for a theatrical performance (taking everything personally makes any clown funnier), it's a good idea to discover what is actually personal to you and what is not. Not everything is personal. Most of life, society, corporations, governments, the culture at large and the world at large doesn't give a fuck about the person—these agencies are impersonal by nature. Distinguish yourself or be extinguished. Knowing what not to take personally means not taking most things personally.

COURTSHIP COMPULSION AND POWER LOSS

Courtship Compulsion ravages the energetic body of the soul and its psychic home, the imagination. This complicated power drain occurs with any excessive emotional investment in an idealized image of the "dream lover," and/or any obsessive search for "The One," the "soulmate" or "twin flame." When these projections are imposed onto any external person who somehow matches that psychic image of the "dream lover" (what Carl Jung calls "the Anima" in men and the "Animus" in women), we can become as psychic vampyres merging with the energy of another in a misguided attempt at achieving "oneness" or some new-age ideal of "alchemical tantric unity." Give me a break; it takes two distinct individuals to sustain any honest interaction and relating.

This power drain also taxes the imaginal faculties that might find more productive and creative outlets through Art, Poetry, Music, Dance, Theatre, Cinema, etc. The power of Venus that's projected onto dream lovers is the same energy fueling Art projects. Without creative outlets, all that psychic energy can backfire and implode into a downward spiral of self-destruction. Courtship compulsion takes tremendous psychic energy to sustain itself and leaves us emotionally drained, always wanting and always needy. It's not courtship itself, which can be a lovely ritual in budding romances, that drains our power. The problem is this one-sided obsession that occurs in our own heads with very little to show for itself beyond the power loss it creates. Courtship compulsion turns into a dumb-down spiral of diminishing returns.

Courtship Compulsion veils a sophisticated ritual of self-torment where love is always wanted but never truly found. The mass culture of advertising controls the Courtship Compulsion by the Beauty Myth oppressing every woman and man mistaking glamour for true beauty (see *The Beauty Myth* by Naomi Wolf). Glamour casualties are assimilated into a vapid world of appearances that drains the dreaming power with the negative spirits of Envy and Greed, the endless comparisons with others, and the endless hungry ghost search for approval, acceptance and love.

Often times, this Courtship Compulsion mythologizes unconditional love. When we seek and expect unconditional love from another person, it places them under tremendous pressure to deliver the impossible. What flawed human person can love unconditionally all the time? This external projection of unconditional love may mask an unmet spiritual need for the love of God, perhaps

the only true source of unconditional love. As this projection persists, we can easily fall into a Poor Baby life where
any kind of love we receive or expect never measures up.
We become snagged in a web of constant disappoint-
ments. If we can trace this projection back to the spiritual
frustration, we may discover how we are love at essence.
When we become the love we seek, the worldly search for
love ceases. Realizing this spiritual truth, we can enjoy
romantic liaisons and endure long term loving relations—
not from any desperate need or search for love but—from
an offering of *self as love* where being in love takes on new
meaning—*to be love is to be in love.*

AN ABORIGINAL VISION OF DREAMING

As these habits of power loss are minimized or elimi-
nated, we may notice a new kind of energy and feeling
inhabiting our lives and relations. Calling this "the power
of dreaming" was inspired by my 1986 encounter with
Guboo Ted Thomas, an Aborigine Koori elder. Guboo
views the planet itself as this massive dreaming entity that
dreams all its inhabitants into existence, the birds, insects,
animals, trees, flowers, fishes, and yes, humans. When I
heard Guboo talk like this, my big white mind freaked out
and threw up a wall thinking, this old guy's batshit crazy.
But there was something about his presence that got under
my skin and relaxed the mental grip I had on thinking I
knew what reality really was.

*Had I unwittingly stumbled into some kind of aborigi-
nal initiation ritual?* Looking into his eyes, I started feeling the presence of the dreaming power of the planet that

he was talking about. And the longer he spoke, the more I felt the dreaming power. And then, he stopped and started singing. I don't remember the words he sang as much as how the energy or spirit in his song zeroed in on my heart, cracking it open. My tears flowed. He smiled and said, "The best is yet to come."

After meeting with Guboo (I interviewed him for a local paper in Boulder CO), I soon became aware of my habits of power loss, namely the Poor Baby and Courtship Compulsion. It wasn't until I diminished their hold on me that I was able to start realizing my dreams...writing books, creating theatre, making films. There was some start and stop over the next few years, including a painful divorce from my first wife, but once I got clear on these power drains my dreams started to come true. I won't bore you here with a list of my accomplishments (check my websites for that). I can say that the rituals and methods in this book were designed to restore the power of dreaming and the insurrection of the Poetic Imagination. When the imagination, the canary in the cultural coal mine, goes belly up the soul soon follows; imagination death precedes death of soul.

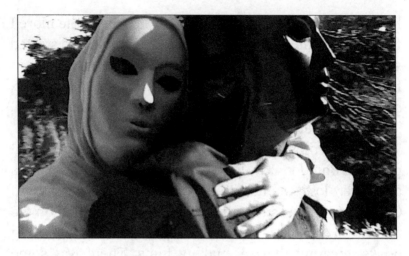

"Shadowplay"
(2017; a short film by Antero Alli)

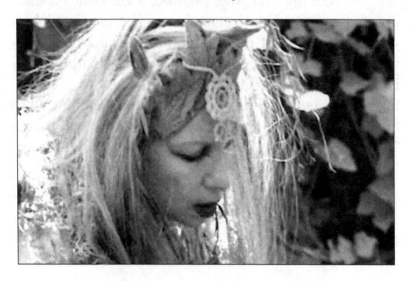

Sylvi Alli in "dreambody/earthbody"
(2012; a paratheatre video document
by Antero Alli)

THE FRUITION OF PERFORMANCE

TOWARDS THE END OF AN ERA

CHRONOLOGY OF THIS WORK

Since 1977 this paratheatrical group work has occurred primarily in non-performance "labs" focusing on method and training, without an audience or any witnesses beyond myself as the Facilitator. Most of these labs met twice a week for eight to ten weeks at a time, sometimes longer, in Berkeley CA (1977–82), Boulder CO (1983–88), Seattle WA (1989–93), again in Berkeley CA (1996–2015) and Portland OR (2016-2019). Between 1977 and 2019, only seven paratheatrical productions were staged in the San Francisco Bay area—*"Coronation at Stillnight"* (1977), *"The Conjunction"* (1978), *"Chapel Perilous: Dreaming Phases for Lovers"* (1982–83), *"Hungry Ghosts of Albion"* (1999), *"Orphans of Delirium"* (2004), *"Songs as Vehicles"* (2004) and *"Requiem for a Friend"* (2005)—and from Autumn 2016 to Winter 2018, five additional productions were staged in Portland.

THE PORTLAND PRODUCTIONS, 2016 to 2018

Each of these five productions were preceded by a 10-week Lab where the sources and rituals were chosen and developed with participants and the final performances directed by myself. *A Turbulence of Muses* (text by Arthur Rimbaud), premiered December 2–4, 2016 to full houses. Our next performance ritual, *Bardoville* (text by Charles Bukowski), premiered May 12–14, 2017 to critical acclaim from Oregon ArtsWatch. Our following production, *Soror Mystica: Ritual Invocation of the Anima* (text by Hilda Doolittle aka HD) premiered December 1–3, 2017 (also to critical acclaim from Oregon ArtsWatch). Our fourth production, *Fallen Monsters* (text by William Blake) premiered May 11–13, 2018 and our final paratheatrical production, *Escape from Chapel Perilous* (text by Sylvia Plath) premiered Nov 29–Dec 2, 2018. All five productions were staged at PerformanceWorks Northwest, Portland and documented on video; links, reviews, & descriptions can be found at:

http://verticalpool.com/paratheatre.html

FROM RITUAL INTO THEATRE

This transition from non-performance oriented ritual experiments into full-blown productions staged before a live audience upset traditional expectations about what constitutes "theatre". Our paratheatrical approach cured the "new performers" from trying to please or impress the audience. They were not there to entertain or to enlighten, but to fully participate in *a total act of offering of the self*. Their total commitment to their visceral and spiritual resonances (with the given sources of the ritual they were performing) emanated a strong force of presence rippling out into the audience. This was no linear theatre experience with a clear narrative line. What was being performed was *a living ritual* dressed up in poetry, live music, projected film sequences, costumes, make-up. Billed as *intermedia performance rituals,* poetry was the only text used and always spoken or sung as oblique narratives, not delivered as any kind of "poetry reading." For example, in "Fallen Monsters" (May 2017) William Blake's poems were arranged and sung as songs by Sylvi Alli. In the December 2018 production of "Escape from Chapel Perilous", poems by Sylvia Plath were delivered as "sermons" in a haunted chapel by Ed Welsh as "Father Timeless". Though the themes, poetry, music and costumes changed with each production, the vital current running through them all was *insurrection of the Poetic Imagination.*

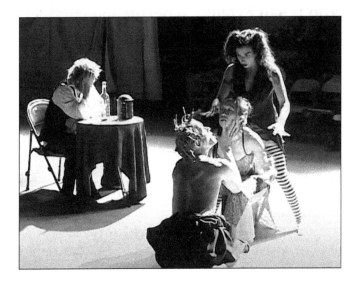

"Orphans of Delirium"
(2004; San Francisco performance/video)

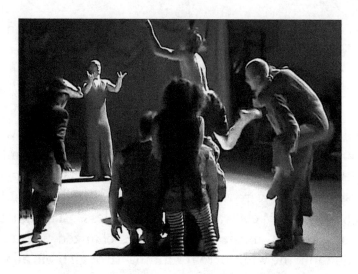

"Orphans of Delirium"
(2004; San Francisco performance/video)

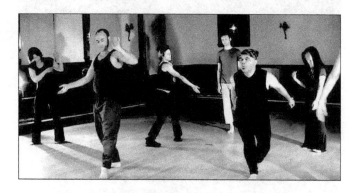

"dreambody/earthbody"
(2012; Berkeley Lab/video)

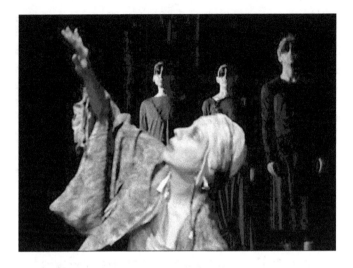

**Sylvi Alli in "A Turbulence of Muses"
(2016; Portland OR performance/video)**

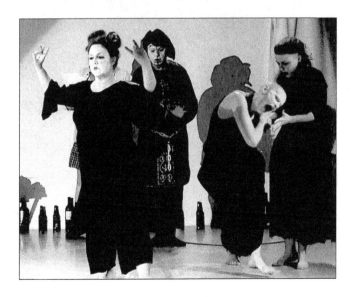

**"Bardoville"
(2017; Portland performance/video)**

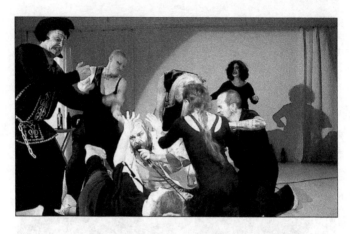

"Bardoville"
(2017; Portland performance/video)

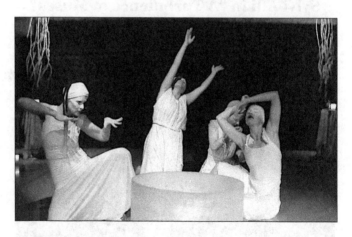

"Soror Mystica: Ritual Invocation of the Anima"
(2017; Portland performance/video)

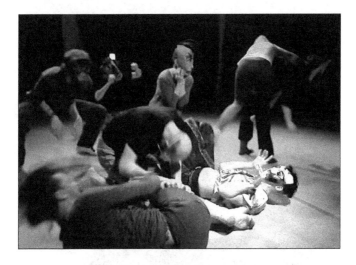

"Fallen Monsters"
(April 2017; rehearsal for Portland performance)

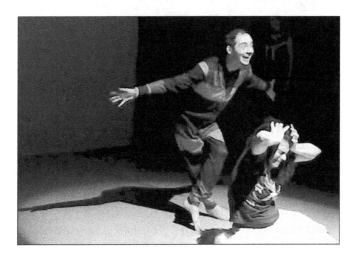

"Fallen Monsters"
(May 2017; Portland performance)

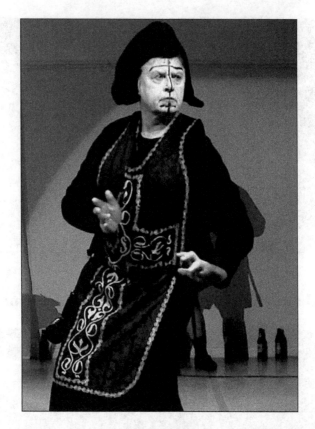

Antero Alli as the Murderous Priest
"Bardoville" (2017; Portland performance)

*With ritual design/theatrical direction by Antero Alli, Bardo-
ville displays elements of classical tragedy/drama such as
confrontation/conflict/resolution. The flow from scene to scene
retained a narrative integrity around which each character
acts and reacts like jazz soloists departing and returning to a
melodic structure and interactive core.*

— Mitch Ritter for Oregon Arts Watch

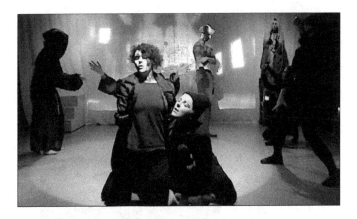

"Escape from Chapel Perilous"
(2018; Portland performance/video)

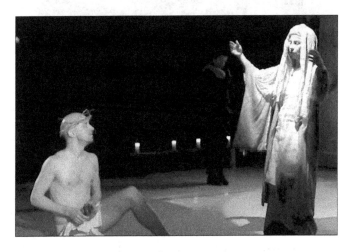

"Escape from Chapel Perilous"
(2018; Portland performance/video)

ABOUT THE AUTHOR

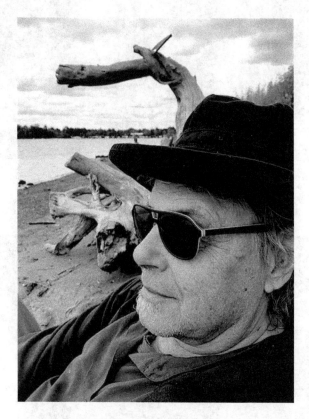

In 1977, Antero was inspired by the Paratheatre of Jerzy Grotowski to create his own paratheatrical medium which has been documented in three of his books, *All Rites Reversed* (Falcon Press, 1987), *Towards an Archeology of the Soul* (Vertical Pool, 2003) and *State of Emergence* (Falcon Press, 2020), plus numerous videos (1991–2018), and by Professor Nicoletta Isar at the Institute of Art

History, Copenhagen University. Between 1977 and 2018, Antero wrote, directed and/or performed in a series of experimental theatre productions. Between 1995 and 2020, Antero wrote and directed twelve feature-length art films—including *The Greater Circulation* (2005), a critically acclaimed cinematic treatment of poet Rainer Maria Rilke's "Requiem for a Friend" and his tribute to French Surrealist, Antonin Artaud in *The Invisible Forest* (2008). He currently resides near a forest in Portland, Oregon with his wife, Sylvi where they play and record music, and make movies.

You can follow Antero at http://verticalpool.com

THE *Original* FALCON PRESS

Invites You to Visit Our Website:
http://originalfalcon.com

At our website you can:

- Browse the online catalog of all of our great titles
- Find out what's available and what's out of stock
- Get special discounts
- Order our titles through our secure online server
- Find products not available anywhere else including:
    - One of a kind and limited availability products
    - Special packages
    - Special pricing
- Get free gifts
- Join our email list for advance notice of New Releases and Special Offers
- Find out about book signings and author events
- Send email to our authors
- Read excerpts of many of our titles
- Find links to our authors' websites
- Discover links to other weird and wonderful sites
- And much, much more

Get online today at http://originalfalcon.com

CPSIA information can be obtained
at www.ICGtesting.com
Printed in the USA
LVHW080111290721
694014LV00013B/834